'Was Sigmund Freud's animosity toward religion just a personal whim, like his fondness for cigars; or was it a commitment to the "scientific naturalism" that is, or should be, essential to psychoanalysis as a discipline? Tamas Pataki, a philosopher well-informed about psychoanalysis, offers a full-throated defense of the latter view, in the process delivering trenchant critiques of representatives of what he argues is a regrettable resurgence of religious thinking in some contemporary psychoanalytic circles. Many analytic superstars, including Winnicott and Bion, take some hard hits. This unapologetic book will surely provoke both plaudits and pushback'.

Robert A. Paul, *Charles Howard Candler Professor of Anthropology and Interdisciplinary Studies at Emory University, Director of the Emory University Psychoanalytic Institute and author of* Our Two Track Minds: Rehabilitating Freud on Culture.

'This book is a delight. Rarely have I enjoyed myself so much reading a work of non-fiction. Erudite with a dry wit, Pataki wears his extensive learning lightly and provides a real service in cutting through conceptual muddle in difficult and obscure texts with an admirable clarity of interpretation and exposition. While he is not shy to excoriate psychoanalysts where they show plain disregard for the facts established by other disciplines, he is equally always ready to acknowledge insight and highlight truth where he finds it. Highly recommended.'

Michael Lacewing, *Senior Head of Department and Head of Psychology at Christ's Hospital School, and formerly Honorary Reader in the Psychoanalysis Unit at University College London, Vice Principal at Heythrop College, University of London, and joint editor with R. Gipps of* The Oxford Handbook of Philosophy and Psychoanalysis.

'This book offers a rigorous and intellectually uncompromising examination of the growing spiritualization of psychoanalysis. With clarity and philosophical precision, Pataki defends explanatory discipline against metaphysical inflation. This is a timely and important intervention for scholars of religion, culture and psychoanalytic theory'.

Tair Caspi, PhD, *Senior Clinical Psychologist in private practice, faculty member in the advanced program for psychoanalytic psychotherapy at Tel Aviv University, previously lectured in the doctoral program in Hermeneutics and Cultural Studies at Bar-Ilan University and author of* Metaphors in Psychoanalysis and co-editor of The Routledge International Handbook of Psychoanalysis and Philosophy.

Psychoanalysis and Religion

In this illuminating volume, Tamas Pataki critically examines Freud's psychoanalytic approach to religion, tracing its intellectual evolution and impact on contemporary theories and practice.

This book delves deeply into Freud's psychoanalytic critique of religion, offering readers a comprehensive analysis of his naturalist perspective and its implications for understanding religious belief systems. Pataki explores Freud's theories alongside the contributions of other prominent thinkers such as Erich Fromm, Ana-Maria Rizzuto, W. W. Meissner, W. R. Bion and N. Symington highlighting their expansions and critiques of Freud's work. Examining Rizzuto's research on God representations, Meissner's insights into the spiritual dimensions of religion, contributions from attachment theory and the emerging trends of spiritually sensitive psychoanalysis and psychoanalytic mysticism the book provides a philosophically rigorous and nuanced comparison of psychoanalytic approaches to religion. This book offers a rich tapestry of ideas that explore the complex interplay between psychology, culture, and spirituality.

Ideal for scholars, students and professionals in psychoanalysis, philosophy, theology and psychology, this book is a valuable resource for anyone seeking to understand the complex relationship between religion and the human psyche.

Tamas Pataki is a philosopher and senior honorary fellow at the University of Melbourne, Australia. He is the author of *Religion, Narcissism and Fanaticism* (2024) and *Wish-fulfilment in Philosophy and Psychoanalysis: The Tyranny of Desire* (2014).

Routledge Introductions to Contemporary Psychoanalysis

Series Editor: Aner Govrin
Executive Editor: Yael Peri Herzovich

Dreams and Dream Interpretation: A Contemporary Introduction
Christian Roesler

Interpersonal Psychoanalysis: A Contemporary Introduction
Anna Maria Loiacono

Psychodynamic and Psychoanalytic Supervision: A Contemporary Introduction
Christine Driver

Couple Relations: A Contemporary Introduction
Mary Morgan

The Oedipus Complex: A Contemporary Introduction
Poul Rohleder

Psychoanalytic Film Theory: A Contemporary Introduction
Ben Tyrer

Thomas Ogden: A Contemporary Introduction
Ofrit Shapira-Berman

Online Psychoanalysis: A Contemporary Introduction
Haim Weinberg

Psychosis: A Contemporary Introduction
Franco De Masi

Free Association: A Contemporary Introduction
Barnaby B. Barratt

Interpretation: A Contemporary Introduction
Aner Govrin

The Negative: A Contemporary Introduction
Rakefet Efrat Holzer

Harry Guntrip: A Contemporary Introduction
Loray Daws

Gender: A Contemporary Introduction
Oren Gozlan

Traumatic Narcissism Theory: A Contemporary Introduction
Daniel Shaw

Philip Bromberg: A Contemporary Introduction
Anthony Bass, Velleda C. Ceccoli

Antisocial Personality Disorder: A Contemporary Introduction
Jessica Yakeley

Pierre Janet: A Contemporary Introduction
Giuseppe Craparo

Psychoanalysis and Religion: A Contemporary Introduction
Tamas Pataki

For more information about this series, please visit: www.routledge.com/Routledge-Introductions-to-Contemporary-Psychoanalysis/book-series/ICP

Psychoanalysis and Religion

A Contemporary Introduction

Tamas Pataki

Routledge
Taylor & Francis Group
LONDON AND NEW YORK

Designed cover image: © Michal Heiman, Asylum 1855–2020, The Sleeper (video, psychoanalytic sofa and Plate 34), exhibition view, Herzliya Museum of Contemporary Art, 2017

First published 2027
by Routledge
4 Park Square, Milton Park, Abingdon, Oxon OX14 4RN

and by Routledge
605 Third Avenue, New York, NY 10158

Routledge is an imprint of the Taylor & Francis Group, an informa business

British Library Cataloguing-in-Publication Data
A catalogue record for this book is available from the British Library

ISBN: 978-1-032-83300-2 (hbk)
ISBN: 978-1-032-82750-6 (pbk)
ISBN: 978-1-003-50870-0 (ebk)

DOI: 10.4324/9781003508700

Typeset in Times New Roman
by Taylor & Francis Books

Contents

Series Editor's Preface

Aner Govrin

Routledge Introductions to Contemporary Psychoanalysis is one of the most prominent psychoanalytic publishing ventures of our day. The series' aim is to become an encyclopedia of psychoanalysis, with each entry given its own book.

This comprehensive series illuminates the intricate landscape of psychoanalytic theory and practice. In this collection of concise yet illuminating volumes, we delve into the influential figures, groundbreaking concepts, and transformative theories that shape the contemporary psychoanalytic landscape.

At the heart of each volume lies a commitment to clarity, accessibility, and depth. Our expert authors, renowned scholars and practitioners in their respective fields, guide readers through the complexities of psychoanalytic thought with precision and enthusiasm. Whether you are a seasoned psychoanalyst, a student eager to explore the field, or a curious reader seeking insight into the human psyche, our series offers a wealth of knowledge and insight.

Each volume serves as a gateway into a specific aspect of psychoanalytic theory and practice. From the pioneering works of Sigmund Freud to the innovative contributions of modern theorists such as Antonino Ferro and Michael Eigen, our series covers a diverse range of topics, including seminal figures, key concepts, and emerging trends. Whether you are interested in classical psychoanalysis, object relations theory, or the intersection of neuroscience and psychoanalysis, you will find a wealth of resources within our collection.

One of the hallmarks of our series is its interdisciplinary approach. While rooted in psychoanalytic theory, our volumes draw upon insights from psychology, philosophy, sociology, and other disciplines to offer a holistic understanding of the human mind and its complexities.

Each volume in the series is crafted with the reader in mind, balancing scholarly rigor with engaging prose. Whether you are embarking on your journey into psychoanalysis or seeking to deepen your understanding of specific topics, our series provides a clear and comprehensive roadmap.

Moreover, our series is committed to fostering dialogue and debate within the psychoanalytic community. Each volume invites readers to critically engage with the material, encouraging reflection, discussion, and further exploration.

We invite you to join us on this journey of discovery as we explore the ever-evolving landscape of psychoanalysis.

Aner Govrin

Preface

The story I tell here of the psychoanalytic engagement with religion is about an arc of decline extending from the intellectual rigor of Freud's writings on religion – while recognizing his errors and omissions – to the drift toward the religious, the mystical, the omnibus of the spiritual that has excited some contemporary psychoanalytic writers to describe their discipline as a religion and its practice as holy. My account of this development is expository but critical, and occasionally combative. It is not the only story that could be told. Other authors have already provided quite different accounts of the same subject and they can speak ably for themselves. The psychoanalytic literature on religion is large and the relevant philosophical and anthropological literature is immeasurable. No individual, certainly not the present writer, could master it. The questions that religious belief and practice raise for anthropology, philosophy and psychoanalysis cut deep. Moreover, as might be expected, there is no one dominant psychoanalytic ethos or attitude to religion in relation to its truth value, therapeutic usefulness or moral and political effects. So for these reasons I have had to be selective, though in a way that I hope still captures the essential features of the development I am calling an arc of decline. Some influential writers were easy to exclude. Jung, Lacan, and Kristeva are excluded since they are remote from this book's concerns. Several scholars, noted in the text, I would have liked to discuss in greater detail, but the want of space did not permit it. In the end I chose what seemed to me some milestones. And because Freud's views have receded in the minds of many psychoanalysts, are ill-understood and misrepresented, I have tried to give a fairly detailed account of Freud's atheism, his ontogenetic and phylogenetic accounts of religion, and his attitudes to religion.

Freud's views are the subject of Chapter 1. Freud set the agenda for the psychoanalysis of religion and he continues as its dominant figure. Most religions have metaphysical and epistemological presuppositions. Most of them make claims about supernatural beings and about what constitutes evidence or reasons for believing in them. Freud understood that psychoanalysis was unable to assess the truth of these claims but could, in light of its understanding of the wishful character of mind, cast a skeptical eye on them. He was able to explain in naturalistic terms how individuals in infancy acquire religions, and, much less persuasively, how the institutions of religions, their practices and dogmas, relations to morality and social structure, evolved. Attachment theory has made important contributions to the understanding of religiosity and religion, and one of its principal doctrines is here contrasted with Freud's ontogenetic account to shed light on both. If naturalistic theories along Freudian lines (or other naturalistic lines) succeed, then supernatural explanations for religion, with their inscrutable claims, become superfluous. Freud also initiated a critique of religion's intellectual and moral vices that has altered Western civilization. He persistently located psychoanalysis as a theory of mind in the federation of the natural sciences, and he worried that without those connections his discipline might become an isolated gnosis in the world of learning.

Chapter 2 discusses the contributions of William Meissner and Ana-Maria Rizzuto. Their extended critiques of Freud, his character traits and his views, shed much light on our subject but are, in the main, rejected. There remained many gaps in Freud's architecture, of course, and these two essentially orthodox psychoanalysts are among those who have filled some of them. Their important positive contributions to the understanding of religiosity are expounded. The influence of Donald Winnicott on these investigators is considered and criticized.

Chapter 3 takes up the views and influence of Erich Fromm. The beginning of the arc of decline is located here in Fromm's indifference to critical distinctions, often wild generalizations and innocence of the history of Western philosophical thought. We substantiate these stern assessments. A careful definition of religion is set out to serve as a metric for the extravagant definitional claims to come.

Chapter 4 selects Neville Symington as the most able representative of the view that psychoanalysis is a spiritual endeavor and, indeed, a religion, albeit a scientific religion. We trace the moral, philosophical and mystical paths that lead him and others to this remarkable conclusion. Many rough patches are exposed. His moral and metaphysical arguments and his reliance on mystical insight are demonstrated to be unsound. Some of Wilfred Bion's philosophical claims, which influenced Symington and other writers who take up similar lines of thought, are briefly but harshly criticized.

The final chapter sets out the narrative pressed by enthusiasts for spiritually sensitive psychoanalysis. It then brings reality into the picture by casting in a brutal light the mass resurgence of religion and spirituality that they appear to acclaim. We conclude that the trend under discussion is essentially a recurrent strategy for regulating the narcissistic economy by means of identifying with powerful supernatural figures or revolving in their orbit.

I have little to say about therapy. It seems to me that sympathetic entertainment of a patient's religious beliefs, as of his or her other beliefs, has always been the gold standard for therapists – it certainly was Freud's, *vide* the case of the *Wolfman* – in whatever light they viewed a loss or openness to religious belief subsequent to treatment. But the new trend asks for more: not only that mystical, religious, and spiritual beliefs, and their alleged benefits be better received or appreciated in the clinic, but that they be granted intellectual as well as clinical respect. Glimmers of this trend can be traced to the 1940s, but waves also appeared after the 1980s. By then, Eastern winds had swept over the West and 'New Age' spirituality with its baubles and superstitions captured the imaginations of many. It seems likely that in the current climate of irrationalism and contempt for science and learning, in the ruinous religious nationalism of the United States, Russia, India, Iran and many other nations, that the trend toward mysticism and nebulous, religiously tinted, spiritualities will continue, and not only in psychoanalysis. I hope that what follows will confirm my negative assessment of these developments and that readers will persist in finding out whether I have succeeded.

I trained as a philosopher, not as a psychoanalyst, and I try to write as a philosopher would with particular regard to the logic of arguments and scrutiny of the evidence for whatever contentions are on the table. We should not believe without reason. When argument or evidence is unsound the conclusion is also likely to be unsound. My reliance on quotation may be unseemly. It is done because sometimes, as with Freud, a matter is expressed so immaculately that it cannot be bettered. At other times, the matter is so confused, so at variance with accepted science or commonsense, that my exposition without backing would appear incredible. The quotations are the evidence on which the expositions are grounded. It was inevitable, given the nature of the subject that the discussion dips into philosophical issues of some complexity. I hope that I have succeeded in making the issues intelligible and in bringing into play some of the vast philosophical literature that bears on them.

Acknowledgements

I wish to thank Professor Aner Govrin, who invited me to write this book and whose suggestions then helped me to improve it. I also wish to express my appreciation of the expeditious helpfulness of all the editorial staff at Routledge and in particular the unfailing judgement of my copy editor Martin Pettitt.

Chapter 1

Sigmund Freud

The young atheist

Psychoanalytic approaches to religion begin, of course, with Sigmund Freud. The psychoanalysis of religion is that borderland where psychoanalysis engages various religious traditions and theologies but must also engage with philosophy, which for more than two millennia has considered the nature of the gods, the reasons for believing in them and the religions devoted to them. All religions have a metaphysics, an account of their gods or spirits or supernatural processes; they all have an epistemology, some account of how the supernatural beings or processes can be known. In considering religions it is impossible to evade their philosophical dimensions. It is unsurprising then that to understand Freud's views on religion he must be located in the philosophical context in which he considered religion. That context we now call 'scientific naturalism', 'materialism' as it used to be called, and the atheism it entails. In fact, Freud's naturalism underlaid everything that he wrote.

Freud passed through life, as Ernest Jones in his great biography said, a 'natural atheist' who had never believed in a supernatural world: he was an atheist before psychoanalytic discovery confirmed him as such. Strictly speaking an atheist is one who denies the existence of gods, but in the course of time the denial of all supernatural beings and processes – spirits, demons, souls, gremlins, mystical experience, reincarnation and so forth – has been shuffled under the rubric. Atheism has ancient roots. Socrates' near

DOI: 10.4324/9781003508700-1

contemporaries – Anaxagoras, Democritus – were notorious for atheism and Socrates himself, though no atheist, was executed in 399 BCE on a trumped-up charge of failing to acknowledge the city's gods (Whitmarsh 2015). On any traditional understanding of personal (human-like) gods, most of the major figures in philosophy since the 17th century have been atheists or deists; the latter usually accepting a First Cause, though not one with personal characteristics. The European Enlightenment was dotted with thinkers hostile to traditional religion and, as Peter Gay and other commentators have insisted, Freud was in several respects directly descended from Voltaire, Diderot, Hume, Kant and Feuerbach (Gay 1987, 1989). It may be noticed at the outset that atheism as such does not entail hostility to religion. Napoleon is said to have remarked that we *need* religion so that the poor should not murder the rich. But for Freud, as we shall see, religion was not only false but an enemy.

Freud declared himself an atheist well before the positivist medical education of 19th-century Vienna had the opportunity to work on him. He famously described himself to his friend Silberstein in 1874 as 'a godless medical man and empiricist'. By 1875 he had read the atheist philosopher Ludwig Feuerbach and wrote to Silberstein, in beguiling contrast to his later disdain for philosophy: 'Among all philosophers I worship and admire this man most' (Gay 1987, 53). The publication of Feuerbach's *The Essence of Christianity* (1989 [1841]) produced a sensation. The idea of the Christian God, he argued, is an involuntary projection of human properties, and humanity comes to self-knowledge by contemplating these projections. Feuerbach detailed how Christian conceptions of divinity derive from aspects of human personality. Therefore, theology is essentially anthropology and the task of reason 'amounts to the destruction of an *illusion* – an illusion, however, which is by no means insignificant but whose effect on mankind, rather, is utterly pernicious' (quoted in Gay 1987, 55). Feuerbach's later work, with which Freud may also have been familiar, derives divine properties from the characteristics of nature as well as humankind. Gods are now seen as products of the various wishes and needs arising from 'the drive-to-happiness': 'gods are those beings that can fulfil and realize those wishes' (Harvey 2013, 144). Freud echoes some of these themes early in his work, as when he writes in the *Psychopathology of Everyday Life*:

> I believe in fact that a great part of the mythological view of the world, which reaches far into most religions, is *nothing other than the psychological process projected into the outer world* … One could venture to explain in this way the myths of paradise and the fall of man, of God, of good and evil, of immortality, and so on, and to transform *metaphysics* into *metapsychology.*
>
> (Freud 1901b, 258–259)

The theme of religious illusion will reappear with greater force in his major critiques of religion more than two decades later.

During 1874 Freud attended lectures by the theist philosopher Franz Brentano, who introduced him, as best one can make out, to variations of the traditional cosmological, ontological and design proofs of the existence of God.[1] Freud was initially impressed by Brentano, 'a genius' and 'fine fellow', and he was troubled by the proofs Brentano set out (Rizzuto 1998, 149–151). The dalliance with theism, however, was brief. In 1875 he visited Manchester and while there read the British empiricists and scientists, Darwin, Huxley, Tyndal, J. S. Mill and, very likely, David Hume. Returning, he wrote again to Silberstein. 'I am more distrustful of philosophy than ever' (Gay 1989, 31). The impact of the empiricists was dramatic, and Freud was doubtless receptive in any case because of the anti-metaphysical, empirical or experimental approach to science and the arts then dominating Vienna's intellectual climate.[2] By the time Freud returned from Manchester he was a principled atheist with a thoroughgoing suspicion of the kind of *a priori* metaphysics to which Brentano had exposed him. References throughout his work show that he was soon aware that Hume, Kant, Feuerbach, Darwin and others had dismantled the scaffolding that held the metaphysical arguments in place. He now understood claims for the existence of supernatural beings as claims to be settled by scientific investigation, not armchair philosophizing, let alone invocation of mystical or religious experience. As he wrote later: 'scientific work is the only road that can lead us to a knowledge of reality outside ourselves' (Freud 1927c, 31).

Some commentators have challenged this undisturbed picture of Freud's atheism. Ana-Maria Rizzuto has done so at length (Rizzuto 1998). She argues that after encountering Brentano Freud had to 'wrestle' with religion because of his inability to refute Brentano's 'scientific proofs'. Freud had been stumped by Brentano: 'Metaphysics could prove God's existence, and Freud lacked the talent to refute Brentano's arguments' (Rizzuto 1998, 153–154). So, instead of refutation Freud had to invent metapsychology to replace metaphysics. This conjecture simply underrates the profound impact that the science of the day and cultural context had on Freud: what Rizzuto thinks is pained recoil from Brentano's proofs is in reality attraction to science and skeptical rejection of their metaphysics. Rizzuto is impressed by an apprehensive passage in a letter to Silberstein, 'Unfortunately, when we allow the God concept we start down a slippery path'. Rizzuto asks insinuatingly: 'How did he conceive of the danger of belief?' (Rizzuto 1998, 151). Her question misconceives Freud's reference to 'the God concept'. She appears to believe that the young Freud was struggling with his God-image, in the sense of that term (discussed below) that has made her own work famous. A better guess has Freud alluding to the 'ontological argument' that Brentano taught him. In crude form, the argument purports to prove the existence of God from the fact that we possess a *concept of a perfect being*, i.e., God; existence is a perfection; therefore, God must exist. The argument can be traced back to St. Augustine and has been reprised in many sophisticated shapes since. It tantalizes and the young student would have been tantalized. In my experience, students introduced to the argument usually feel that wool is being pulled over their eyes, react initially with intrigue and eventually contempt. The young Freud probably did much the same. It seems most likely that his encounter with Brentano shaped, not his fear of religion as Rizzuto believes, but the contempt for *a priori* philosophizing that he later liberally expressed. Rizzuto also finds deep significance in another passage of banter with Silberstein supposed to show Freud's struggle with his adolescent religiosity. Freud wrote that he had lost the fear of 'the envy of the gods' (Rizzuto 1998, 148ff). The concept is not Biblical (so far as I know) and could hardly have been invented by an adolescent. But rather than being revelatory of religious turmoil the reference is surely to the concept of *phthonus*, the envy of the gods, prominent in the Greek tragedy that Freud and Silberstein were then studying. Adolescent banter may reflect deep concerns, of course, but often enough just cleverness in schoolwork. Finally, Rizzuto boldly accuses Freud of lying about his knowledge of Hebrew; knowledge of Hebrew, she surmises, suggests a deeper immersion in religion than Freud was willing to avow. Freud said late in life that he had never understood the language, but Rizzuto says that he must have because he was taught Hebrew and his father inscribed in Hebrew the precious Bible he gifted to Freud; he would scarcely have done so, Rizzuto reasons, had he believed that Freud would be unable to read his heartfelt thoughts (Rizzuto 1998, 77). Rizzuto and several other critics who make similar claims seem unaware that children in secular Jewish families are often taught to recite but not necessarily to understand Hebrew. Pronouncing the holy words is the critical thing, not comprehension, rather as in the Latin Mass, which no-one but the priest (if he) can understand. The residues of word-magic endure. (My father also inscribed intimate Hebrew texts in our prayer books, knowing that we children couldn't understand them.) It is notable that Freud did not have a bar-mitzvah, a time when most Jewish boys do confront the issues of religious identity and belief in the supernatural and are often compelled to study at least the rudiments of Hebrew. It seems that Rizzuto's conjecture that Freud had once struggled with religion, leaving a deforming cast upon his later thought, has little to support it.

Scientific naturalist

In a chapter of his *New Introductory Lectures on Psychoanalysis* (1933a), 'The question of a *Weltanschauung*', Freud explains that if '*Weltanschauung*' is meant to denote an encompassing world view 'which solves all the problems of existence uniformly on the basis of an overriding hypothesis', provides answers to every pressing question and invests security in life, then psychoanalysis emphatically does not have a *Weltanschauung*.

> As a specialist science, a branch of psychology – a depth psychology or psychology of the unconscious – it is quite unfit to construct a *Weltanschauung* of its own: it must accept the scientific one … Apart from this it is marked by negative characteristics, by its limitation to what is at the moment knowable and by its sharp rejection of certain elements that

> are alien to it. It asserts that there are no sources of knowledge of the universe other than the intellectual working-over of carefully scrutinized observations – in other words, what we call research – and alongside of it no knowledge derived from revelation, intuition or divination.
>
> (1933a, 158–159)

Freud goes on to emphasize that psychoanalysis, like all science, is 'a program, the fulfilment of which is relegated to the future' (1933a, 158–159).[3] Several features of the outlook expressed in these passages are essential for understanding all of Freud's work, but especially for understanding his views on religion. Freud was an *empiricist*, holding that all knowledge is ultimately based on sense experience or observation. Other presumptive sources of knowledge, including religious or mystical experience are spurious. He does not discount the possibility of innate knowledge, 'primal phantasies' for example, but these he thought are based ultimately on primeval experience.

Later in the chapter, Freud distinguishes psychoanalysis as a general theory of mind, as a method of inquiry and as a therapy. And he came to think, perhaps unexpectedly, that the first of these was paramount. In 1928 he wrote to his friend Oskar Pfister:

> I have often said that I hold the purely medical importance of analysis is outweighed by its importance to science as whole, and that its general influence by means of clarification and the exposure of error exceeds its therapeutic value to the individual.
>
> (Freud 2023 [1963], 120)

Psychoanalysis as a method of treatment is, of course, not a science, though it should be informed by science and adopt the caution of science. Because psychoanalysis sits in the federation of the sciences – or so Freud hoped it would – it should *as a method of investigation and as a theory of mind* adopt scientific methods. Here, it is important to observe a distinction in the German language. Overlooking it has caused confusion about the scientific status of psychoanalysis within psychoanalytic discourse and beyond it. Freud believed that psychoanalysis had not only a place in systematic inquiry and knowledge (*die Wissenschaft*), usually translated as 'science', but is also broadly continuous with the adjacent exact or natural sciences (*die Naturwissenschaft*), that is to say, physics, biology, physiology and such neuroscience, psychophysics and experimental psychology as there was in his time. This view is explicit in many passages:

> Analysts … cannot repudiate their descent from exact science and their community with its representatives … Instead of waiting for the moment when they will be able to escape from the constraint of the familiar laws of physics and chemistry, they hope for the emergence of more extensive and deeper-reaching natural laws, to which they are ready to submit. Analysts are at bottom incorrigible mechanists and materialists, even though they seek to avoid robbing mind and spirit of their still unrecognized characteristics. So, too, they embark on the investigation of occult phenomena only because they expect in that way finally to exclude the wishes of mankind from material reality.
>
> (Freud 1941d [1921], 178–179)

In a typical reminder, he writes: 'we must recollect that all our provisional ideas in psychology will presumably some day be based on an organic substructure' (1914c, 78). In contemporary terms, Freud was a scientific *naturalist*: only natural causal entities and natural causal powers exist, and natural science – physics fundamentally – tells us what these are.[4] The naturalist denies that there are non-natural or supernatural entities, powers or processes.[5] Some naturalists include the mental in the natural world, but Freud seems to have been, as the passage above suggests, also a *physicalist* or, to render his view to his time, a *materialist*. It is difficult to gauge his commitment to fully reductive materialism. His views on the relation between the mental and the physical remained unresolved – which is unsurprising since the matter is still unresolved. The most plausible attributions to him are a tight form of *mind-brain parallelism* or *dual-aspect monism*. [6] On the second construal, mental states are identical to physical states; on the first, they supervene on them: on neither view can the mental separate from the physical: mental states cannot *fly free* of physical states of the brain.

Here then is the crucial bearing of these seemingly remote ontological matters on Freud's views about religion: gods, spirits and souls conceived to be immaterial thinking things independent of material states are impossible; insofar as (most) religions are interlaced with such conceptions they must be false. It follows, too, that if occult phenomena in which the mental *is* supposed to fly free do exist then the naturalistic hypothesis is disconfirmed.

Now, Freud was, of course, the great investigator of mental life. How does the materialism imputed to him sit with what he regarded as his distinctive contribution, 'precisely in having extended research to the mental field. And … without such a psychology science would be very incomplete' (1933a, 159). How does his commitment to the mental square with the reductive materialism, 'the medical materialism' that was in the air he breathed even before he began his medical studies? The answer goes something like this. In his scientific training Freud absorbed the best tenets of the science of his day, which are still the best tenets of science: careful observation; formulating and testing hypotheses and discarding falsified ones; seeking consilience and simplicity; recognizing that scientific progress is piecemeal and, at its frontiers, provisional or corrigible – open to correction. Religion, at least most scriptural religion, is of course a very different kettle of fish. At the time Freud entered the laboratories, medical materialism was making immense strides by treating human beings as material systems devoid of vitalistic, immaterial or spiritual elements. The scientists at the forefront of this biophysics movement included Freud's teachers and colleagues, men such as Ernst Brücke and Theodor Meynert, following in the footsteps of giants such as Herman Helmholtz. Freud often testified to their immense influence. 'Brücke', he affirmed, 'was the greatest authority that worked upon me' (Gay 1989, 33). Excepting a few pockets of Romantic psychiatry it was generally agreed by the mid-19th century that all mental illness was a disease of the central nervous system. That view shaped Freud's earliest approaches to psychotherapy (Freud 1954 [1887–1902]). However, as his interest shifted from patients' central nervous systems to their interpersonal experiences his views began to cross the dominant psychiatry. Freud insisted on the role of emotions and, of course, sexual desire. He realized that he could neither treat nor understand his patients without employing the ordinary language of common-sense psychology: of wishing, belief, fear, fantasy, jealousy, anxiety and so forth.

> Like other neuropathologists, I was trained to employ local diagnoses and electro-prognosis, and it still strikes me myself as strange that the case histories I write should read like stories and that, as one might say, they lack the serious stamp of science ... The fact is that local diagnosis and electrical reactions lead nowhere in the study of hysteria, whereas a detailed description of mental processes such as we are accustomed to find in the works of imaginative writers enables me, with the use of a few psychological formulas, to at least obtain some kind of insight into the course of that affection.
>
> (1895d, 160–161)

This understanding did not lead Freud to abandon the view of psychological processes having neurobiological foundations, eventually explicable in neurobiological terms. Instead, the apparently incompatible commitments to reductive materialism and mental causation expressed in the indispensable idiom of common-sense psychology created a split in his theorizing between the quasi-neurological framework of his metapsychology and an augmented mentalistic psychology, sometimes referred to as the clinical theory. The early attempt in the *Project for a Scientific Psychology* (1954 [1887–1902]) of creating an entirely materialistic psychology was largely deferred, not abandoned. Freud left the matter hanging, but his many later excursions into metapsychology show that he clearly hoped for a future mapping of clinical theory onto neurobiology. That may be impossible, for complex reasons of principle, but today we know that fruitful psychoanalytic theoretical work proceeds on both the neurobiological and clinical planes.

That is where we must leave Freud's basic ontology. Its implications for the understanding of religion are profound. Scientific naturalism precludes supernatural entities such as gods or spirits and supernatural processes. There may be intrinsic value in undergoing religious, mystical or spiritual experiences – they may have therapeutic benefits – but insofar as they claim access to supernatural knowledge, their claims must be fallacious. There are no supernatural sources of knowledge because there is no supernatural domain. Since scientific naturalism incorporates psychoanalysis, psychoanalysis is incompatible with supernatural religion. Freud wrote to Pfister in 1929: 'Analysis produces no new world view. But it does not need one, for it rests on the general scientific world view with which the religious one remains incompatible' (Gay 1987, 81). This is no idle matter for religion or other spiritualities, including those wishing to forego the name of religion. Scientific naturalism is the most comprehensive and explanatorily rich 'big picture' we have of our universe. Since scientific naturalism is flatly incompatible with religions and spiritualities that posit supernatural entities or processes, a heavy burden of proof weighs on the latter.

The naturalistic accounts of religion

I have been highlighting the scientific-naturalistic context of Freud's atheism because it is the critical circumstance for understanding his approach to religion. As could be expected, there is no dearth of suggestions about his personal motivations for being an atheist, and some of these are discussed below. But for now we turn to the details of the naturalistic theories of religion that Freud developed. Naturalism frames the problematic of religion this way. Most religions are intricated with conceptions of supernatural beings, gods or spirits, but there are no such beings, so what's going on? How is it that human beings from earliest times have conceived, feared and worshipped them? And how were the institutions, rites and doctrines of the various religions initiated and preserved when they are in reality built on sand? Freud provided naturalistic answers to these questions or, more precisely, outlines of answers. If successful, then they strengthen the case for naturalism because supernatural intervention to explain religious phenomena is rendered superfluous.

Freud believed with most anthropologists of his day that religion was aptly characterized as belief in one or many spiritual beings and the various other beliefs and practices that arise in connection with them. Not all spirits are objects of worship or veneration; often, they are objects of fear, but when they are worshipped they are called 'gods' and devotion to them is called 'theism'. Freud was expressly concerned with the Judeo-Christian tradition or, as he says indifferently, the 'religion of the Western peoples' or 'present-day white Christian civilization', and he focuses deliberately on what the 'ordinary man understands by his religion'. Freud knew something of Islam, Eastern religions and non-theistic systems of spirituality, claiming the title of religion, but his published remarks on these are few.[7] It is often objected that Freud chose a 'definitional strategy' that intentionally narrowed the concept of religion to fit his theories while excluding non-theistic spiritualities such as certain expressions of Buddhism, pantheism and (anachronistically) the spiritual strivings under the head of New Age Spirituality.[8] The objection misses the mark. Freud did not 'choose a definitional strategy'; he supposed, correctly, that the concept of religion could not be extracted from its historical (indeed, prehistorical) and conceptual context as belief in spiritual (or supernatural) beings together with the rituals, offerings and so forth, associated with them. That is the anthropological paradigm that fixes the concept.

The ontogenesis of religiosity

It is useful to divide Freud's account into parts. This section is concerned with his ontogenetic theory: the motives and means by which a person acquires the dispositions and concepts that constitute their religiosity. The next part concerns the role of phylogenesis in sustaining individual religiosity and in the establishment of religion as a cultural institution. Later in the chapter we consider Freud's attitudes to religion and some of the criticism his views have attracted.

Freud's *tour de force, The Future of an Illusion* (1927c), begins unexpectedly with a dense, somber and puzzling account of the emergence of civilization or culture.[9] Civilized life, Freud says, inevitably requires renunciation of instinctual pleasures, and since such renunciations are painful every individual becomes 'virtually an enemy of civilization'. Moreover, because masses are lazy, unintelligent and lacking fondness for work, every civilization is built upon coercion by a minority, entailing further restrictions on instinctual pleasure. But then, if civilization is as burdensome and contrary to our natural dispositions as Freud suggests, why did it arise in the first place? Freud answers that the benefits outweigh the costs. Civilization may be an enemy to the individual, but there is another, more formidable enemy: Nature, which

> destroys us – coldly, cruelly, relentlessly … It was precisely because of [the] dangers with which nature threatens us that we came together and created civilization … For the principal task of civilization, its actual *raison d'etre*, is to defend us against nature. (1927c, 15)

Civilization has achieved a great deal for humanity, he continues, yet the inevitable confrontations with nature constantly revive the feelings of weakness and helplessness experienced as severe blows to our 'natural narcissism': 'Man's self-regard seriously menaced, calls for consolation: life and the universe must be robbed of its terrors', and man's curiosity must be satisfied (1927c, 16).

Humanity takes a first step toward religion by humanizing nature: if everywhere in nature there are Beings around us of a kind that we know in our own society, then we can breathe freely, can feel at home in the uncanny and can deal by psychical means with our senseless anxiety. (1927c, 17)

Now, the introduction of spirits at this point, for reasons that will become evident, is unexpected, and a brief digression is required to explain it. Earlier in *Totem and Taboo* (1912–1913) Freud argued that spirits are in effect projections of human personality or souls.[10] So far as the humanization of nature goes, Freud mostly followed his great anthropological predecessors. Edward Tylor, the father of British cultural anthropology, contended that belief in souls and spiritual beings was the earliest religion; he named it 'Animism'. Tylor considered the invention of the concepts of *soul* and *spirit* momentous intellectual or philosophical achievements. With these concepts, many enigmatic phenomena could be explained: the difference between living and dead bodies, between being awake and asleep, natural causation, and so forth. The anthropomorphic character of the spirits and the greatest of the gods, reflecting the dispositions of human souls has a tremendously important consequence: the supernatural world of gods and spirits becomes an extension of the human social world. Freud agreed that the Animistic doctrine of spirits was a kind of theory or philosophy, a solution to enigmatic problems, especially the problem of distinguishing life and death. But he did not agree that intellectual problems were the main issue. Typically, he focused on the underlying emotional conflicts. He agreed with those who say that:

> the first-born spirits were *evil* spirits, and who derive the idea of the soul from the impression made by death upon the survivors. The only difference is that we do not lay stress on the intellectual problem with which death confronts the living; in our view the force which gives the impetus to research is rather to be attributed to the emotional conflict into which the survivors are plunged.
>
> (Freud 1912–1913, 92–93)

The emotional conflict concerns ambivalence toward the dead. While writing *Totem and Taboo* Freud was preoccupied with the obsessional neuroses, and he believed that primitive man shared with neurotics the heightened ambivalence and belief in the omnipotence of thought that are striking features of the neurotic condition. With the loss of an ambivalently loved figure, the bereaved person projects his anger to keep the memory a loving one (1912–1913, 59–63, 91–94).[11] This explained, Freud reasoned, the primarily demonic character of spirits and the constant demand for propitiating them. At this stage Freud had not yet explored the phenomenology of mourning, as he was shortly to do, but he is now able to explain the origin of spirits (of the conception of *spirit*), as a conjecture engendered not by philosophical curiosity but by emotional necessity. 'Spirits and demons', he says, 'are only projections of man's own emotional impulses. He turns his emotional cathexis into persons, he peoples the world with them and meets his internal mental processes outside himself' (1912–1913, 92, 61–63). What are these 'emotional cathexes'? Although he is as yet unable to articulate the thought explicitly, the projections must be of cathected ('charged') objects or self-representations (or of 'internal objects', as we shall later say, in the sense Melanie Klein has given the term). To function as spiritual, person-like beings they must have personal identity, and not just be unresolved galaxies of emotions. The projection of object and self-representations eventually comes to play an indispensable role in Freudian accounts of the dynamics of religiosity. Most striking, however, is the second shift of perspective Freud effected. Feuerbach had argued that the gods are projections of human personality. Freud provided the motivation by showing that the projections were in service to the ineluctable need for *human* relationship. At heart, relationship to the spiritual or divine is essentially driven by the need to maintain human relationship.

Returning to the discussion of *Future of an Illusion*. Freud next observes that the helplessness felt in relation to the humanized spirits now inhering in nature is a repetition of a prototype of infantile dependence on parents, most of all on the powerful father. And so it is natural that the inspirited forces of nature should be experienced not only as person-like agents but also be imparted *the specific character of the father*. Freud has arrived at his subject, monotheism: God is modeled on fathers. An early statement is important for its rare departure from an almost exclusive focus on the father and for squarely placing religiosity in the context of biological dependency.

> Psychoanalysis has made us familiar with the intimate connection between the father-complex and belief in God; it has shown us that a personal God is, psychologically speaking, nothing other than an exalted father, and it brings us evidence every day of how young people lose their religious beliefs as soon as their father's authority breaks down. Thus, we recognize that the roots for the need for religion are in the parental complex; the almighty and just God, and kindly Nature, appear to us as grand sublimations of father and mother, or rather as revivals and restorations of the young child's ideas of them. Biologically speaking, religiousness is to be traced to the small child's long-drawn-out helplessness and need for help.
>
> (1910c, 123)

By the time of *Future*, mother's role in religious formation has almost vanished, and Nature is no longer 'kindly' but lethal. Both shifts are curious. Freud knew that the mother who satisfied the infant's primary needs is also his first love object and protector. He insisted that a child's need for protection motivates the turn to religious objects, but mother's protection, he now says, is 'soon replaced by the stronger father, who retains that position for the rest of childhood' (1927c, 24). Freud knew that something was amiss. The hasty shift to the 'stronger father' is inconsistent with his own developmental principles: for Freud, 'deeper' usually means 'earlier'; and his attempts to explain the emergence of matriarchal religions in the historical record and the ubiquity of female divinities are self-consciously awkward (1912–1913, 1939a). It seems probable that personal factors and patriarchal influence on a mind even as original as Freud's partly account for these lapses. But there is a more important motive hidden in the logic of Freud's larger thesis. We will see in the section below that Freud needed to coordinate his ontogenetic account with what he considered to be one of his great discoveries, the foundation of religion based on the murder of the 'primal father', the alpha male of the primitive human horde who becomes the phylogenetic prototype of God. To fully account for the depth and profundity of religion, Freud reasoned, required a synergistic combination of revived memory traces of that archaic parricide with images of the actual father saturated with ambivalent oedipal feeling. The individual's image of God based on the latter had to merge with the inherited memory traces of the primal father, the original God (1923d, 85). Mothers had no part to play in that momentous union and were therefore peripheral to the religious disposition. Suffice to say here that Freud's neglect of pre-oedipal dynamics was an error, though perhaps an unavoidable one, and the argument from phylogenesis has less appeal today than in Freud's Vienna. But we are running ahead.

What, then, is the ontogenetic theory? 'The psychical origin of religious ideas', Freud says,

> are not precipitates of experience or end-results of thinking: they are illusions, fulfilments of the oldest, strongest and most

> urgent wishes of mankind. The secret of their strength lies in the strength of those wishes … [T]he terrifying impression of helplessness in childhood aroused the need for protection – for protection through love – which was provided by the father; and the recognition that this helplessness lasts throughout life made it necessary to cling to the existence of the father, but this time a more powerful one. Thus, the benevolent rule of a divine Providence allays our fears of the danger of life; the establishment of a moral world order ensures the fulfilment of the demands of justice, which have often remained unfulfilled in human civilization; and the prolongation of earthly existence in future life provides the local and temporal framework in which these wish-fulfilments take place. Answers to the riddles that tempt the curiosity of man, such as how the universe began or what the relation between body and mind, are developed in conformity with the underlying assumptions of this system. It is an enormous relief to the individual psyche if the conflicts of its childhood arising from the father complex – conflicts it has never wholly overcome – are removed from it and brought to a solution that is universally accepted.
>
> (1927c, 30)

This is an attractive statement, not least because it explains quite fully the similarities between the wishful expectations placed on a benign father and on divine Providence. But how exactly does Freud derive the illusional character of religious ideas from the unquestionable premise of infantile dependency and – let us go along with Freud here – the need for father's protection? Freud defines illusions *prescriptively* as wish-fulfilling beliefs caused by wishes. This is neither the ordinary conception of illusion (magical, optical illusions, mirages, vain hopes) nor whatever it is that Winnicott later made of it (creative imagination, perhaps). An illusion is a *belief:* it may be or become true. The middle-class girl who wishfully believes she will marry a prince may find her prince. Freud says of religious doctrines that:

> all of them are illusions and insusceptible of proof. No-one can be compelled to think them true, to believe in them. Some

> of them are so improbable, so incompatible with everything we have laboriously discovered about the reality of the world, that we may *compare them – if we pay proper regard to the psychological differences – to delusions.*
>
> (1927c, 31; my italics.)

Delusions are defined in this framework as beliefs that are caused by wishes, contradict reality, and are immune to rational revision. Since Freud believed that religious beliefs are false and held dogmatically and irrationally his considered view is that religious beliefs are *delusion-like*, although not delusions.[12] We know why he thought religious beliefs were false: the supernatural claims of religion are incompatible with scientific naturalism; the traditional justifications offered for religious doctrines are scandalously muddled and unworthy of belief (1927c, 26–29); and he believed, although he doesn't make much show of it, that philosophers and scientists had knocked out the pins supporting religious doctrines by refuting the traditional philosophical arguments for the existence of God. The falsehood of theism is not a psychoanalytic finding, but psychoanalysis contributes to its undermining. Freud's ontogenetic account does not formally contradict theism. As Freud says, the truth-value of religious doctrines is outside the scope of psychoanalytic doctrines 'but it is a very striking fact' that religions represent the world 'exactly as we are bound to wish it to be' (1927c, 33). The contradiction is found in the larger epistemological frame: between the simplicity and fertility of the naturalistic account of the world and the religious picture relying on incomprehensible notions of incorporeal, creative agents and questionable epistemology.

Suppose that religious beliefs are indeed false. Nevertheless, how can Freud be certain that they are caused by wishes? Maybe they are just unmotivated mistakes? Maybe they are the accidental byproducts of evolutionary processes, as Richard Dawkins (2006) holds? Why was Freud certain that religious beliefs were not just false but illusions? To answer this key question requires some preparation, for Freud's account is rather more complex than appears at first sight.

> When the growing individual finds that he is destined to remain a child forever, that he can never do without protection against strange superior powers, he lends those powers the features belonging to the figure of his father; *he creates for himself the gods* whom he dreads, whom he seeks to propitiate, to whom he nevertheless entrusts his own protection. Thus his longing for a father is a motive identical with his need for protection against the consequences of his human weakness. The defense against childish helplessness is what lends its characteristic features to the *adult's reaction to the helplessness which he* has to acknowledge – a reaction which is precisely the formation of religion.
>
> (1927c, 24; my italics)

Freud knew, of course, that most people are born into religions and that only some become religious: religious ideas are presented ready-made as 'the heritage of many generations' (1927c, 21). So, when he says that individuals 'create gods' for themselves it would be more accurate to say (in the monotheistic context) that they *shape* the culturally given conceptions of God, in the first instance on the model of their (idealized) fathers. In other words – that Freud oddly does not use in this context – the child's paternal images or representations (or, better, internal objects, as I shall soon say) are *projected* into the cultural image of God, which is then experienced as a real father. Freud says: 'the god of each … is formed in the likeness of his father … at bottom God is nothing other than an exalted father' (1912–1913, 147). Elsewhere, he underlines the transformation: '[God] really is the father' (1933a, 163). It seems clear that Freud is affirming more than that God symbolizes or represents the father: God *is* a surrogate father. It would seem useful to adopt Hanna Segal's distinction between *symbol* and *symbolic equation* to explicate the identity God = father that Freud is striving after (Segal 1986). Then we can distinguish between 'mere' object representations or images and those that are concretely experienced as internal objects. We can then say that internal objects, and not just representations, are projected into the cultural images of God. Thus in the devoutly religious person the unconscious equation God = father is not merely representational or symbolic, it is experienced as a reality.

The projections in question must be unconscious. Relating to God as if to a father is sometimes encouraged, especially in Christian cultures, but the identity Freud insists on – that father and God are at heart one and the same – must remain repressed, otherwise the entire project of theistic belief would unravel. Now, there is a difference between infantile wishes for solicitude preserved in the unconscious, and conscious adult wishes that are similar but stem from realistic, adult appreciations of life's adversity. We know that an adult's wishes for protection and love can be satisfied by religious devotion, as it can be in other ways. Identifying with, or living in the orbit of the powerful, whether a political leader, an ethnic group or nation, may provide a sense of security, of mattering, of being loved. Freud's deep insight is that infantile repressed wishes directed at father may also be satisfied in the self-same relation, albeit in a roundabout manner that he designates 'wish-fulfillment' or 'substitutive satisfaction'.[13] *Unconscious* infantile wishes, whose object is father's solicitude, may be satisfied *at the same time as* adult wishes stemming from realistic dependent needs and anxieties directed at God. In the devout, those in whom religion goes deep, the relationship to God is not a sequel to an earlier relationship with father; it is a current relationship with a projected paternal internal object: *it is as if* the relationship to God is a relationship (in unconscious phantasy) with a concrete idealized father. This fact (if it is a fact) explains a great deal. It is the reason why some people experience religious devotion so profoundly, poignantly and yet precariously, requiring regular 'turning inwards' or reconnection in prayer, sacrifice and self-abasement. It is the reason why Freud believed that analysis of the oedipal fixation to father would contribute to dissolving religious attachments. Dissolving the attachment to the father imago is tantamount to dissolving the attachment to God. It also explains why he thought that religion could protect against neuroses (1927c, 85). One element of an internal conflict, which Freud considered a precondition of neurosis, the menacing paternal internal object (a component of the superego), is projected into the external world and so defuses the internal conflict – there to cause havoc in the field of social pathology.[14]

We now come to the crucial reason why Freud was convinced that religious beliefs are not just false but wishfully engendered. How are we to conceive the unconscious wish-fulfilling relationship with God-experienced-as father? As we saw, Freud emphasizes that psychology is unable to determine the truth or falsity of religious beliefs. But he observes the remarkable coincidence that these beliefs should represent matters just as we would wish them to be. They certainly *look* like wish-fulfilling beliefs, and Freud had a powerful overarching theory about that; in fact, one of the most important theories in psychoanalysis: that of wish-fulfillment. Wish-fulfillment may appear to play a lesser role in contemporary psychoanalysis than it has in the past. That is not really so. In classical psychoanalytic theory most mental disorders were considered largely as pathologies of desire and conflict, of wishes or other id-motivational states in conflict with reality or ego and superego. That has given way in contemporary theory to a dominant concern with pathologies of developmental deficit resulting from environmental, attachment or interactional failure. Speaking generally, psychoanalysis *appears* less concerned with the pathology of desire than of belief – or various belief-like structures – internal working models (Bowlby), representations of interactions generalized (D. N. Stern), and so on. The attention to environmental deficiency and early impairment creates the impression of diminished interest in the desiderative, conflictual and wish-fulfilling aspects of mind. But in fact, that theoretical contrast is unstable. Trauma, privation, deprivation are measurable only against a backdrop of need and desire, and the language of object or interpersonal relations is otiose without reference to mutual desiderative and affective relations. So, in reality motivational notions remain key, and Freud's notion of wish-fulfillment reappears in different guises, as omnipotent phantasy, projective identification, manic defense, actualization (J. Sandler), and related ways of conceptualizing illusional or delusional constructions.

The illusional – or wish-fulfilling – theory of religion achieved an impressive consilience between religious beliefs and practices, the much larger class of wish-fulfilling phenomena, and the underlying metapsychology:

> the principal function of the mental mechanism is to relieve the individual from the tensions created in him by his needs ... But the satisfaction of ... part of these needs ... is regularly frustrated by reality ... The whole course of the history of civilization is no more than an account of the various methods adopted by mankind for 'binding' their unsatisfied wishes ... Myths, religion and morality find their place in this scheme as attempts to seek a compensation for the lack of satisfaction of human wishes.
>
> (1913j, 186–187)

Recall the main thesis of *The Interpretation of Dreams* (1900a): all dreams, neurotic symptoms, daydreams and unconscious phantasies are wish-fulfilments or attempted wish-fulfilments. To these, Freud soon added delusions, hallucinations, jokes, some art, motivated slips, magical or omnipotent thinking, morality and religion. That all these superficially unrelated phenomena shared the distinction of being roundabout ways of fulfilling wishes struck Freud as a remarkable unification and corroboration of his scientific research. Freud's conception of wish-fulfillment or *substitutive* or symbolic satisfaction is an innovation, a new concept with a resemblance to an established one. Very briefly, then, in the established or ordinary conception of wish-fulfillment: a person wishes for something; they get it; they know or believe that they get it and, as a consequence, cease wishing for it. Their wishing ceases because they *believe* that they got it: and it is *because* they get it that they believe that they got it: one could come to believe that one won a lottery by being knocked on the head with a mallet, but that would not count as wish-fulfillment. Finally, it doesn't matter on this conception whether a wished-for object is attained by personal effort or by gift. On the novel *technical notion* that Freud introduced, the person does *not* get what they wish for, the *real* objects of the wish are not attained, only a substitute or semblance is, *viz.* a dream, hallucination, meaning-bearing symptom or belief that what is wished for is indeed so. Characteristically, either the wished-for state of affairs does not occur or, even if it does, it has no causal role in the cessation of the wish. Speaking broadly, human action is terminated by belief states, not exhaustion. Usually, only belief, or an experiential state like a dream functioning informationally like a belief, has a causal role in suspending or pacifying a wish – more or less temporarily. So, Freud writes that a dream

> does not simply give expression to a thought, but represents the wish fulfilled as a hallucinatory experience … the dream does not simply reproduce the stimulus [the wish], but removes it, gets rid of it, deals with it, by means of a kind of experience.
> (1916–1917, 129)

The dream is fleeting, but during the dream (and perhaps for some period after) it is *as if* (in the unconscious meaning of the dream) the wished-for state of affairs occurred, and that illusion suspends or pacifies the wish. Freud was able to show with impressive success that processes along these lines operate in the broad range of phenomena listed above.

His insight can be generalized this way. If the world cannot be altered by action to accord with our wishes, then, in certain circumstances – of sleep, reverie, regression, dissociation, projective manipulation – we manage to alter our *beliefs* about it: these beliefs suffice to pacify or suspend ineluctable wishes because they represent the world to us as we would wish it to be; through their prism the world appears more congenial. In Freud's view, then, religious beliefs and the phantasies embodied in rituals can be considered counterfeit evidence unconsciously understood to represent our circumstances as we wish them to be, just like in dreams, hallucinations and symptoms. Thus, Freud saw attachment to God principally as a wish-fulfilling means of keeping alive a relationship to an idealized father deemed essential for safety and security. If that *is* correct, then we have a deep explanation for why, despite the implausibility of religious beliefs and the strangeness of religious practices, people still cling to them tenaciously, treat them with awe and reverence, and may kill if the embedded relationship is threatened.

Finally, it is frequently alleged against Freud, sometimes by people who should know better, as if it were a *reductio ad absurdum*, that he regarded all human dependency as infantile and religious people as particularly infantile and neurotic, if not delusional. William Meissner writes: 'The Freudian supposition … implies that all religious behavior and belief is a form of obsessive-compulsive neurosis. The associations of Freud's descriptions are full of implications of infantilism and superstition' (1984, 58). And Black writes in a travesty that according to Freud's theory it was the 'ignorant and morally pusillanimous people … who were likely to be attracted to religion' (2006b, 3). Freud certainly held that the human is a dependent animal, but he did not think, as the quoted passages from him make clear, that all dependency is infantile. Insofar as the devoutly religious are fixated on, or regressed to, early parental *imagos* or introjects they are infantile. But neither in Freud's view nor in subsequent psychoanalytic clinical writing is this condition understood pejoratively. (Freud occasionally uses the term pejoratively, as when he says of *religion* that the 'whole thing is so patently infantile'). The fixation does not imply that the entire personality is infantile, let alone neurotic. Freud knew as well as anyone that there were religious figures who met the measure of greatness on any scale. In Freud's scheme of things, although all neuroses involve a degree of infantilism, not all infantilisms are neurotic. Perversions, for example, and certain apparently regressed but conflict-free conditions, he did not consider neurotic. Neuroses require a condition of intrapsychic conflict, and Freud did not think that all the religious folk in the world were beset by conflict. Quite the opposite, he thought that religious conviction could obviate individual neurosis: 'devout believers are safeguarded in a high degree against the risk of certain neurotic illnesses; their acceptance of the universal neurosis spares them the task of constructing a personal one' (1927c, 44). Freud often brings neurosis and religion into conjunction but is always careful to distinguish them. He speaks of 'analogy', 'resemblance', 'parallel', 'counterpart' and 'comparison'. His earliest paper devoted to religion concludes: 'In view of these *similarities and analogies* one might venture to regard obsessional neurosis as a *pathological counterpart* of the formation of religion, and to describe that neurosis as an individual religiosity and religion as a universal neurosis' (1907b, 126–127; my italics). Not the religious individual is neurotic, but rather *religion*, in some sort of corporate sense, may be regarded as a universal neurosis. Again, it is not the religious person who may be psychotic but the *dogmas of religion* that 'bear the character of psychotic symptoms but which, as a group phenomena, escape the curse of isolation' (1939a, 85). Freud's thought here is opaque. He seems to have in mind an unstable doctrine about social development of the sort that was common in the late 19th and early 20th centuries. Just as a child passes through stages of infantile neuroses, 'humanity as a whole, in its development through the ages, fell into states analogous to the neuroses' (1939a, 80). Religion as a social phenomenon is a neurosis-like state of humanity. Just how humanity could fall into states analogous to neuroses without individuals acquiring individual neuroses is not entirely clear.

A comparison with attachment theory

It may be helpful at this point to briefly contrast Freud's views with some of the best contemporary work on the psychology of religion. Attachment theorists such as Lee A. Kirkpatrick (1999, 2005) and Pehr Granqvist (2020) have described the conspicuous similarities between infant attachment behavior and the religious adult's behavior. Infants cry and raise their arms to be picked up, adults pray with arms outstretched, beseeching God; infants seek proximity to carers, and adults believe that God is omniscient, always watching; and so forth. However, according to these researchers the similarities are not to be explained by the persistence of infantile wishes but by the fact that the primary attachment behavioral system described by John Bowlby (1971 [1969]) as active from birth remains active in the adult. Granqvist writes:

> Unlike Freud … attachment scholars do not tend to view attachment behavior in adults as manifestations of regression or unhealthy dependency. In contrast, Bowlby not only claimed that the attachment system is active from cradle to grave but he also regarded attachment as healthy throughout the life cycle.
>
> (Granqvist 2020, 88)

Whether that is an accurate description of Freud's views is moot, but the key point to pick up is that attachment theorists don't see the child's relationship to the parent as still alive in the later one; they think that would involve unhealthy regression. In contrast to Freud's view that past mental content is dynamically alive in the present, they see the continuing operation of the attachment system.[15]

It is interesting and important for the psychology of religion that both psychoanalytic and attachment theory are deficient when considered against the full historical arc of religious phenomena. For most of the human record, religions do not manifest a pronounced attachment or communion aspect. The hunter-gatherer and pastoral groups that have managed to remain unaffected by monotheism and so provide a clue to prehistory usually display cool manipulative pragmatism toward their gods and spirits; dependency is ritualized and muted (Horton 1997, 373ff). The idea that the deity should be loved ('with all one's heart, mind and soul') and beseeched for love is a very recent entrant in religious attitudes. The Aristotelian *Magna Moralia* states that a man would have to be eccentric if he claimed to love Zeus, and there are few records in ancient polytheism where attachment to any god could be described as intense or dependent.[16] To be sure, the older religions sought the favor of gods and spirits, propitiated and entreated them, but there were no illusions about gods reciprocating love. Epicurus thought that there may be gods, but they have better things to do than be bothered with us. The gods had to be kept onside. The principle of worship was practical: I give, so you give – rain, wealth, offspring – in return. Freud makes the striking remark that only when a people lose confidence in their ability to influence the spirits and gods do they abandon manipulation, magic and imprecation, and seek relationship based on suppliant dependency (1933a, 165). Mystical or quasi-mystical attempts at building psychological bridges between man and deity appear to peak in times of social distress when ordinary human relations are disrupted. Episodic associations between social insecurity, misery, depressive trends and yearning for personal relationship with gods antedate Christianity, which itself arose in the misery of the 3rd century CE when urban centers of migration failed to provide the previous security of family, clan and locality. People in lonely, impersonal places were ready to accept 'a peculiarly intense parental relationship with a spiritual being – a relationship that had no real parallel in the locally based cults in their earlier lives'.[17] Searching for communion with the gods seems to have arisen in Egypt and Mesopotamia during times of social dislocation in the latter half of the second millennium BCE as the Bronze Age empires collapsed. In Greece, eras of political and social discord gave rise to mystical movements in the 6th century BCE (Pythagoras, Orphism), the aftermath of the Peloponnesian War (Plato) and the third century CE (Plotinus). The most imaginative works of Jewish and Christian mysticism were composed in the darkest times of the Middle Ages (Scholem 1995 [1954]). Increasing dislocation, confusion, despair and the re-emergence of mystical and spiritual yearnings are features of our time also.

The fact that forms of polytheism and spirit-belief still occupy the greater part of the religious spectrum in Asian but also monotheistic religions, as they did historically, is as problematic for the psychoanalytic theories of religion as for attachment theory. They have both focused too exclusively on the Abrahamic and Buddhist traditions. Our understanding of religiosity may be quite different had they not done so.[18] But another significant difficulty confronts attachment theory, one that Freud's account avoids in an illuminating way. Attachment theory struggles to explain how children can form profound affective attachments to non-corporeal figures. Granqvist writes:

> Although infants' and toddlers' use of attachment surrogates is typically directed to concrete objects, from preschool age onward … the child's cast of surrogate objects may come to include a whole new set of abstract, invisible, and non-corporeal characters. Thus, as children experience themselves thinking and planning, and imagine the intentions of their social interaction partners, they may begin to apply their mentalizing ideas to abstract, symbolic – yet typically highly anthropomorphized – others.
>
> (Granqvist 2020, 41)

This statement requires unpacking. It is one thing to think about incorporeal objects such as fictional characters and gods; it is another to endow them with human attributes; and another, still, for these objects to become targets of profound emotion, which is predicated on triggering the attachment system. That last requires the intricate personal interactions, close physical contact, mirroring and repetitive rescue from distress that attachment investigators have made so familiar. How do passive incorporeal objects attract emotion and devotion? It happens. People weep at the death of fictional characters. But we must discriminate. The attachments to fictional or other incorporeal objects – whatever the quality on the attachment spectrum – are *very* different in intensity from intimate human relations, and even at their most intense rarely attain that of attachment to pets. Granqvist's explanation seems incomplete, at best. Freud has a very good explanation: the relationship to incorporeal figures like gods, when it is deep, is essentially the continuation of an unconscious relationship to the father. That explains both the anthropomorphic character of the gods and the modulated intensity of the relationship to them. We know now that matters are more complex than Freud conceived them. The projection of maternal representations into the given cultural matrix is far more significant than Freud imagined, as are projections of self-representations, injecting narcissistic elements into the relationship with God. Other important figures and education (perhaps indoctrination) also enter into the construction of religiosity. However, the *essential architecture* of Freud's ontogenetic account displays more than a little of the truth.

The phylogenetic story

Well before Freud had given the final touches to his ontogenetic account he had been eyeing a larger canvas (1912–1913). He wished to explain not only how individuals acquired religion in the cradle of the family but also the historical origins of religion, of monotheistic religion in particular. Then, as darkness gathered over Europe the deeply rooted theme of his Jewish self-definition led Freud to explore the historical roots of Jewish character and antisemitism. These aims coalesced in the last published work in his lifetime, *Moses and Monotheism* (1939a), one of his most flawed and provocative essays. It was important to Freud that psychoanalysis should not become alienated from humanistic and natural sciences. In biology, anthropology and history he sought both confirmations of psychoanalysis and material for its application. Religion has many rich points of contact. Its supernatural doctrines, strange apparently irrational rituals, its function as a container for individual and group narcissism, its potential to unleash harrowing violence cry out, as it were, for psychoanalytic attention. As was his wont, Freud commenced by peering into the deep past.

Following Darwin, he assumed that our pre-civilized ancestors lived in small polygynous groups dominated by a single alpha male, much like the modern gorilla. In this arrangement the powerful male, the 'primal father', lived with his female consorts and offspring, with exclusive rights to the females; his sons were kept in subjection, banished or killed. He lived, in Robert A. Paul's words, 'by the untransformed imperatives of sex, aggression and narcissism' (Paul 2021, 22). In their unhappy subjection and exile the brothers were disposed to form ties of affection and cooperation based on homosexual feeling. Then, Freud speculates

> One day the brothers who had been driven out came together, killed and devoured their father and so made an end of the patriarchal horde. United, they had the courage to do and succeeded in doing what would have been impossible for them individually. (Some cultural advance, perhaps, command over some new weapon, had given them the impression of strength.) Cannibal savages as they were, it goes without saying that they devoured their victim as well as killing him. The violent primal father had doubtless been the feared and envied model of each one of the company of brothers; and in the act of devouring him they accomplished their identification with him, and each one of them acquired a portion of his strength.
>
> (1912–1913, 141–142; 1939a, 81ff)

The sons hated the tyrant but also loved and admired him; remorse and the wish to undo the murder ensued. To avoid further violent competition to replace the primal father and reestablish autocracy the brothers forged a kind of social compact: they renounced claims upon their group's females and substituted for the murdered father sacred totem animals who were invested with the father's authority and inviolability. The chosen totem animal, Freud says, 'struck the sons as a natural and obvious substitute for the father'. This may seem strange, Freud admits, but not in light of the fact that humankind did not then feel a gulf between themselves and animals, as children do not today (1912–1913, 144; 1939a, 82). It is notable that shamanistic hunter-gatherer groups to this day revere kinship between humans and animals. From the primal murder Freud proceeds to derive the origins of exogamy and totemism, two fundamental features, as he thought, of primitive societies. The argument goes something like this. Intrinsic to totemism, the first religion in Freud's view, are the earliest moral prohibitions or taboos against incest and murder. Taboo against mating within the clan ensured exogamy and therefore obviated incest, and the prohibition by 'deferred obedience' against killing the totem (= the primal father), extended to fratricide and eventually inaugurated the wider prohibition against murder. Freud then closes the circle. The taboos correspond to the fundamental prohibitions against the unconscious wishes of the Oedipus complex – on murdering the father and incest with the mother. So 'the beginnings of religion, morals, society … converge in the Oedipus complex' (1912–1913, 156).

Freud insisted that this convenient outcome was not the consequence of a single prehistorical homicide (1939a, 81ff). The primal murder was not a unique event in human prehistory; revolts against primal fathers by coalitions of sons, sequels of remorse, symbolic restitution and social reorganization were repeated countlessly over unmeasured time. Good. But how do these discrete prehistorical events explain the origins and transmission specifically of religious traditions? Why were the egalitarian compacts more than evanescent blips in the autocratic order? Freud needed to explain how the consequences of the momentous, traumatic primal murders were passed across the generations. Notoriously, contradicting Darwinian evolutionary theory he knew well, Freud invoked the Lamarckian notion of the inheritance of acquired characteristics. Lamarckian theory holds, roughly, that individual or generational experiences can be assimilated into the genotype, and so something like 'memory traces' can be passed on as phylogenetic inheritance. The theory (at least until recently) was rejected in its entirety by geneticists and evolutionary biologists. Freud had vacillated over the years on precisely *what* is preserved as archaic heritage (1912–1913, 31). But at last he decided that

> the archaic inheritance of human beings comprises not only dispositions but also subject-matter – memory traces of the experience of earlier generations … My position, no doubt, is made more difficult by the present attitude of biological science, which refuses to hear of the inheritance of acquired characters by succeeding generations. I must, however, in all modesty confess that nevertheless I cannot do without this factor in biological evolution.
>
> (1939a, 99–100)

Ernest Jones recalls Freud's reaction when asked to moderate this uncompromising view. Freud would say only that the authorities were all wrong (Jones 1957, III, 336).[19] Just how much Freud had staked on the biological transmission of inherited memory traces became clear with the rediscovered 'lost' paper on metapsychology which its editors named 'A phylogenetic fantasy: Overview of the transference neuroses' (Freud 1987) Freud there shows inordinate ambition to combine biological, historical and psychoanalytic propositions into a coherent whole that would, as he said, 'leave his calling card on biology'. As the chosen title of the paper suggests, much of the article is pure fantasy.

Freud had other, clinical reasons for his insistence on the inheritance of acquired characteristics, not just high ambitions, and we shall come to them presently. But for now we press on outlining the phylogenetic story. The devastating experiences and associations of the original oedipal crimes, it goes, are repressed and preserved as memory traces, as an archaic heritage of humanity. In the course of time a kind of social latency intervenes and the original meanings of the ancestors' deeds are forgotten. As with most repressed material, the archaic heritage eventually finds distorted expression. The return of the repressed, and the various means of dealing with it, eventually come to engender social organization, religion and morality. In short, the complicity in the common crime and the brothers' compact underlie cooperative, egalitarian society; religion is fundamentally based on the sense of guilt attaching to the crime; morality is based on the exigencies of society, the need for cooperation and social virtues, so formed, together with the penance demanded by the sense of guilt (1912–1913, 146). Moreover, Freud maintained that nothing but the re-emergence of the archaic heritage rising from the very depths of the unconscious could account for the sublimity, profundity and majesty of religious emotion (1939a, 128). Finally, Freud conceives of a line of religious development from totemism, where the animal totem represents the primal father, progressing to humanization of the totems forming gods still closely associated with animals; then to polytheisms reflecting the fraternal structures of the brothers; and, eventually, through the regressive revival of memories of the primal crime reevoked by the murders of Moses and Jesus he arrived at the formation of monotheistic Judaism and Christianity. Intimacy with the primal father is at last restored.[20] Freud lamely notes that the great-mother goddesses must have appeared somewhere in this process, but has little to say that is persuasive about that countervailing development.

It is impossible in a faint sketch to do justice to Freud's eclectic assimilation of anthropological, historical, religious and psychoanalytic materials. Some difficulties will have already disturbed the reader. Freud reasoned, often cogently, from a number of premises that turned out to be false. He accepted Darwin's speculation about the social structure of early human groups, but the speculation is almost certainly mistaken. Our modern human ancestors probably were organized like our nearer cousins, the chimpanzee and bonobo, who live in large hierarchical multi-male and multi-female groups, permitting a considerable degree of promiscuous mating.[21] He borrowed from J. J. Atkinson the idea that conditions in the primal horde naturally lead to a successful rebellion by the oppressed sons, to killing and eating the primal father, and to their subsequent negotiated exogamy (1912–1913, 126ff). We know now that in chimpanzee and bonobo communities the females, not the young males, leave the group, and it was probably so in early modern humans. Freud thought he had strong confirmation in the work of W. Robertson Smith on totemism. Smith developed an intricate but critically vulnerable hypothesis linking the totem meal to periodic ritual sacrifice, including the oblations of primitive societies and Christian communion. Freud linked this congenial hypothesis to psychoanalytic observations of infant phobias made by himself, Ferenczi, and others, suggesting that the phobic object was in fact the father displaced onto the feared animal. The convergence between Atkinson's hypothesis and the psychoanalytic observations led Freud to believe that he had good grounds for identifying the totem animal with the primal father, and festive totem meals with commemorations of the primal crime. 'Psychoanalysis' he declared, has revealed that the totem animal is in reality a substitute for the father … The ambivalent emotional attitude, which to this day characterizes the father complex in our children and which often persists into adult life, seems to extend to the totem animal in its capacity to substitute for the father. (1912–1913, 141)

Alas, the totemic theory accepted by Freud and many anthropologists at the time was already hanging by a slender thread as Freud was writing *Totem and Taboo*. It soon became evident that totemism is both too confined and too various to serve as the foundation of original religion. Freud was aware of some of these difficulties but chose to ignore them (1912–1913, 109).

Interestingly, evidence of which Freud seemed unaware, the wonderful animal depictions in caves and shelters of the late Paleolithic period, suggest animal worship or, more likely, worship of spirits taking animal forms. An abundance of evidence suggests belief in the immanence of spirits in cave walls, supplication and sacrifice – hallmarks of religion. By the time of the Magdalenian culture (approximately 12,000–17,000 years ago), there were strong indications of shamanism, forms of religion widespread even today (Clottes 2016). Though the parietal art initially might seem helpful to Freud's totemic argument, it is in fact lethal. The preponderance of cave paintings is of animal *prey*; moreover, the acknowledged totems of many clans are vegetables. Neither prey nor vegetables seem befitting the power and sanctity invested in the totemic surrogate of the primal father.

Freud, we said, had clinical reasons for insisting on phylogenetic influence, and these are worth noting. He was arrested by phenomena that seemed inexplicable in terms of the individual's immediate experience and environment. Certain symbols reoccurring in dreams and phantasy appear to be universal, yet unlearned. Moreover, children appear to have a burden of information incongruent with their actual experience. The 'primal phantasies' of coitus and castration, Freud concluded:

> are a phylogenetic endowment. In them the individual reaches beyond his own experience into primaeval experience at points where his own experiences become rudimentary. It seems to me quite possible that all the things that are told to us today in analysis as phantasy – the seduction of children, the inflaming of sexual excitement by observing parental intercourse, the threat of castration (or rather castration itself) – were once real occurrences in the primeval times of the human family, and that children in their phantasies are simply filling in the gaps in individual truth with prehistoric truth.
>
> (1916–1917, 371)

Freud also noted discordance between displayed affect in certain conditions and the presumptive cause. The intense guilt and compulsiveness of obsessional neurotics and some religious people seemed disproportionate to any real experience the subjects may have undergone. To account for the intensity of these feelings, Freud thought, required some relation to real experiences, to 'historical truth', as he awkwardly says. He found the historical truth in the phylogenetic experience of the primal murder, as, of course, he was disposed to do (1939a, 84ff). It would be agreed on all sides today that Freud's observations had merit, but a deeper appreciation of pre-oedipal dynamics might have checked his inclination to trawl through prehistory to find their cause.

Robert A. Paul, in an admirable book (Paul 2021), is among the few psychoanalysts and anthropologists who have rallied to Freud's defense. He argues that Freud probably *was* right about the primal crime: it occurred and re-occurred, over eons, in much the way Freud described and with the consequences he described.

Something like the sequence of primal murder followed by social readjustment into fraternal, more egalitarian structures, and exogamy, explains remarkably well the transition from what were autocratic structures headed by dominant males in the early human hordes to the egalitarian, peaceful and cooperative cultures still observable among hunter-gatherers and some pastoral peoples today. These societies are marked by their extraordinary cooperativeness and allowance for individual autonomy: 'No leaders or chiefs exert their will over others; people do not (normatively) interfere with others or tell them what to do', and major resources are shared (2021, 54). It is a good guess that these social organizations predominated before Neolithic times and the emergence of agriculture, hierarchy and kings. How does Paul explain this transition in terms of the neo-Darwinian synthesis? After repeated rebellions against autocratic males, as Freud describes it, and the repeated establishment of egalitarian, fraternal and cooperative dispensations, genetic traits favoring cooperation, sharing, control of aggressive and dominance-seeking behavior are selected out along normal Darwinian lines. This is most plausible. But we don't yet have an argument for the development of *any* religion, let alone monotheistic religions, which are unknown among hunter-gatherers and pastoralists. Further argument would be required to show that cooperative, peaceful, aggression-inhibiting social structures lead to monotheism; and such arguments have, of course, been attempted, though not along Freudian lines. Without pursuing this line of thought, it may be observed in the light of the violent history of monotheistic religions that tolerance, irenic character and cooperativeness do not stand out.

It would take us too far afield to penetrate into the territory of *Moses and Monotheism*, into Freud's discussion of the origins of monotheism and the formation of Jewish character. Only the briefest description can be attempted of a complex and troubled argument. Freud was seized by his own original ideas but also ambivalent about them. His emotional investment and the grave circumstances in which the book was written doubtless account for the untidiness that all critics have noted. The opening chapters argue that Moses, the central character in Jewish genealogy, was a high-ranking Egyptian associated with the court of the Egyptian king Amenhotep IV (circa 1353–1336 BCE), who changed his name to Akhenaten when he established, albeit fleetingly, the worship of a single creative solar god, Aten.[22] On this telling, Akhenaten was the first monotheist; his monotheism was a high moral doctrine of justice and truth imbibed by Moses, who was determined to promulgate it after the Egyptian priesthood had almost erased it. He chose a Semitic people then resident in Egypt as his vehicle and by sheer force of will imposed on them the worship of Aten, and famously led them out of Egypt. These people were a seminal fraction of those who later became the early Israelites and eventually the Jewish people. Freud accepted the doubtful view of the Biblical scholar Ernst Sellin that after the exodus from Egypt the Israelites rebelled and ungratefully killed Moses. In the course of the exodus, the original Egyptian cohort merged with another Semitic people in the area of Sinai known as Kadesh and adopted their worship of Yahweh, a local, violent and 'bloodthirsty' volcano god. 'This union, from which sprang the people of Israel, found expression in the adoption of a new religion, common to all the tribes, the religion of Yahweh' (1939a, 37). The priest of the local religion, the son-in-law of Jethro, was also called Moses, though a less mercurial character than the Egyptian Moses. So, two Moses of very different character were soldered together in the Biblical account, explaining the many contradictions of character recorded there. After the ferocious conquest of Canaan led by the violent and merciless volcano god Yahweh, a kind of cultural repression and latency set in. Then, with the return of the repressed, on the model of the return of the primal father, the Egyptian Moses came to entirely eclipse the other. The austere god of morality and justice of the Egyptian Moses is slowly revived with the prophets and merges with the image of the great man and the god Yahweh. The reason that a single god became so compelling for the Israelites, Freud continues, was that behind Yahweh stood the solitary figure of Moses and the remorse for murdering him; and behind *that* figure lurked as archaic heritage the memory of the killing of the primal father of the horde: 'When Moses brought the people an idea of a single god, it was not a novelty but signified the revival of an experience in the primaeval ages of the human family which had long vanished from men's conscious memory' (1939a, 129). From there it was a short step, with suitable modifications, to explain the eventual triumph of Christianity, a religion essentially of the Son whose sacrifice was at the same time retribution and absolution for the killing of the primal father. Freud's steps are ingenious, but we cannot follow him further.

Ingenious but untenable. Enough has been said about inherited memory traces to be skeptical of Freud's reliance on them, although as far as the revenant Moses goes it is less derelict than his construction of the primal murder; it is conceivable that if there was indeed such a man his memory would be retained as a *cultural* inheritance retrievable from the storehouse of tradition in despairing circumstances (such as the threat of Assyrian obliteration in the time of the prophets). And in such circumstances the idealization of charismatic narcissistic leaders into Messianic proportions received with 'admiration, awe and gratitude' is not uncommon, as we know all too well. But Freud was at the mercy of historical and archaeological research, and subsequent research has been unkind to his assumptions. Even if it were possible to ignore the inconvenient gulf between the reign of Akhenaten and the timing of the exodus, and even if firm evidence, so far unavailable (Dever 2006), could be found for an exodus led by a man called Moses and the ensuing military conquest of Canaan, there is the problem that Akhenaten's innovations were not as Freud imagined them to be. Recent excavations in Akhenaten's city suggest not monotheism but monolatry, the worship of several gods, with the god Aten favored by the king, and very likely worshipped only by the king, who himself was worshipped. Aten was represented by a solar disk, a representation inconvenient to Freud's claim about the Mosaic prohibition on images leading to greater Israelite capacity for abstraction and intellectuality. The sublime and lofty tone, the emphasis on justice (Ma'at) that Freud found in the religion of Aten, is in fact not very different, if different at all, from that found in the previous millennium of Egyptian hymns and wisdom literature (Bellah 2011). In short, the religion of Aten that Freud conjectured as the basis for Israelite monotheism didn't happen. The first step goes awry, and after that it was misstep after misstep. Freud cleaved so closely to the Biblical account that it did not occur to him that Israelite monotheism may be an outgrowth of Canaanite monolatry, with the triumph of a favored god over others (Collins 2007).

Freud's attitude to religion

Toward the end of his life, Freud wrote, 'Neither in my private life nor in my writings have I ever made a secret of being an out and out unbeliever' (Gay 1987, 38). Atheists are not obliged to deprecate religion. Some atheists endorse institutional religion, recognizing its unifying and potentially therapeutic role. Freud was not an atheist of that stripe; he was resolutely hostile to religion. He wrote to his ecclesiastical friend Oskar Pfister of his 'absolutely negative attitude toward religion, in every form and dilution' (Gay 1989, 527). He believed optimistically that *his* age, having passed through the eras of religion and philosophy, was entering the era of science; whatever usefulness religion once had was superseded. Science would much better bear the burden of explanation, cure and consolation previously borne by religion. But Freud did not believe that science *is* a religion or would replace religion with all its trappings. Few things could have been further from his thoughts.[23]

Freud's objections to religion are mostly of a piece with the Enlightenment critique. Like Hume and Kant, however, he remained in life in the moral harbor of the Judeo-Christian tradition. He objected to religion on moral, practical and intellectual grounds, but his great originality lay in singling out the sexually repressive and aggressive aspects of the tradition – the excessive repression of sexuality, the inherent aggression directed against out-groups, religion's exploitation of guilt feeling, and the stifling of thought associated with religious education. These things he criticized fiercely. Certain moral injunctions and social expectations, such as the command to love thy neighbor or uncompromising conjugal fidelity, he considered unrealistic demands of the 'un-psychological proceedings of the cultural superego'. But given that he came to believe that religious guilt derived ultimately from the primal murder, and aggression ultimately from an inherent death instinct, he could not consistently lay the blame for all the guilt and aggression civilization is heir to at the feet of religion.

The critique of civilization, sexual morality and religion that Freud initiated (1908d, 1921c, 1927c, 1930a, 1933a) and the social impact of his clinical discoveries is well appreciated. They have altered the course of Western civilization. Psychoanalysis has so thoroughly penetrated the understanding of relations between persons, of mental illness and treatment, of anthropology, religion, political and social psychology that its mark has become invisible.

Yet Freud's harshest objections to religion relate not to their part in enforcing rigid moralities, perpetuating aggression and guilt, or even to the error of their doctrines and superfluity of their institutions. The gravamen of his case is that religion cripples the intelligence and detaches it from reality. Freud believed that the foundational doctrines of religions are false and therefore their practices and institutions are built on sand. They misrepresent reality, and so ultimately offend and deform reason. In this, he is at one with a tradition that extends from Lucretius and notably through Hume, Schopenhauer and Nietzsche to many of our contemporaries. We have already noted critical elements specific to Freud's background. They may be repeated here: scientific naturalism is the best big picture of the world we have and the best methodology for exploring it; it is incompatible with supernaturalist religions; there is neither evidence nor other warrant (*a priori* argument, for example) for supposing there are gods or other supernatural beings or processes. Moreover, powerful naturalistic theories, e.g., Freud's theories of religious ontogenesis and phylogenesis explain why it is that, despite the lack of warrant, people – even educated people – embrace religions passionately. These theories do not refute religious belief but contribute to undermining it.

So, poorly warranted and continuously eroded by cultural and scientific advance, Freud argues, religions found it necessary to place an embargo on critical thought. Freud warns that 'the prohibition against thought issued by religion to assist its self-preservation is … far from being free from danger either for the individual or for human society' (1933a, 171). In passages reminiscent of Schopenhauer and Nietzsche he writes that religion survives by instilling 'sweet – or bitter-sweet – poison' into young minds so that

> by the time the child's intellect awakens, the doctrines of religion have already become unassailable … When a man has once brought himself to accept uncritically all the absurdities that religious doctrines put before him and even to overlook the contradictions between them, we need not greatly be surprised at the weakness of his intellect. But we have no other means of controlling our instinctual nature but our intelligence. How can we expect people who are under the dominance of prohibitions of thought to attain to the psychological ideal, the primacy of the intelligence?
>
> (1927c, 48–49)

On the one hand, religious conceptions are incompatible with the naturalistic worldview and, on the other hand, religious worldviews are replete with absurdity, implausibility and contradiction. The latter assessment Freud held independently of his assessment of the merits of scientific naturalism. The content of religious ideology and the manner in which it is inculcated not only affronts the intelligence but draws people into a state of psychical infantilism and mass delusion (1930a, 84–85). Religion detaches the individual from a realistic appreciation of the way the world is, human and natural. The world is no nursery. When Pfister responds with rhapsodic optimism to *Future*'s moral pessimism, Freud is exasperated: 'And finally – let me be impolite for once – how the devil do you reconcile all that we experience and have to expect in this world with your assumption of a moral world order?' (Freud 2023 [1963], 123). When Pfister urges that religion must be higher than science because it is beautiful and noble, salvific and therapeutic, Freud retorts: 'The question is not what belief is more pleasing or more comfortable or more advantageous to life, but of what may approximate more closely to the puzzling reality that lies outside us' (2023 [1963], 133). The whole idea of a Provident religion, he writes:

> is so patently infantile, so foreign to reality, that to anyone with a friendly attitude to humanity it is painful to think that the great majority of mortals will never be able to rise above this view of life. It is still more humiliating to discover how

> large a number of people living today, who cannot but see that this religion is not tenable nevertheless try to defend it piece by piece in a series of pitiful rearguard actions. One would like to mix among the ranks of believers in order to meet these philosophers, who think they can rescue the God of religion with an impersonal, shadowy and abstract principle.
>
> (1930a, 74)

Freud is acidulous about the authors of these 'rearguard actions', the philosophers and crypto-mystics. They are capable of 'every possible sort of dishonesty and intellectual misdemeanor'. They stretch the meaning of words until nothing is left of their original sense and 'God' becomes the name of some vague principle.

Critics persist in describing as 'deeply religious' anyone who admits to a vague sense of man's insignificance or impotence in the face of the universe, although what constitutes the essence of the religious attitude is not this feeling but only the next step after it, the reaction which seeks a remedy for it. (1927c, 32)

Freud prefers the old dogmatists, who are at least straightforward folk. To Marie Bonaparte, he wrote:

> You are right: one is in danger of overestimating the frequency of an irreligious attitude among intellectuals. I get convinced of that just now on observing the reactions to my [*Future of an*] *Illusion*. That comes from the most varied drinks being offered under the name of 'religion', with a minimal percentage of alcohol – really non-alcoholic but still they get drunk on it … The old drinkers were a respectable body.
>
> (Gay 1987, 12)

Gay comments that Freud thought 'getting drunk on apple juice was nothing less than ridiculous'. Freud, one imagines, would have been horrified by the inebriated 'spirituality' that we discuss below.

Some of the disreputable rearguard are forerunners of postmodernist tincture that Freud labeled 'intellectual nihilism'. His targets are not entirely clear. Perhaps he had in mind Henri Bergson or Hans Vaihinger or William James. Postmodernism is a jumble, but broadly speaking it repudiates the notion of an objective standpoint from which the world can be viewed; there are no objective facts to which our true beliefs correspond; there is no indubitable foundation for knowledge; there is no one way the world is, there are only 'local truths' conditioned by local cultures, practices, interests, interpretations and perspectives. That's quite a diverse package, to be sure, but Freud gets close to the nub of the matter. He characterizes his targets as abrogating what he calls the criterion of truth: correspondence with reality.[24] If there is no such criterion, he avers, then 'all opinions are equally true and equally false. And no-one has a right to accuse anyone else of error' (1933a, 176). If there are no facts, then it is all the same what dose of morphine a patient is administered, and 'if there were no such thing as knowledge distinguished among our opinions by corresponding to reality, we might build bridges just as well out of cardboard as out of stone' (1933a, 176). Freud aptly refers to the ancient liar paradox (of Epimenides). To adapt it: if what the postmodernist says is true, then it is not true, because then there is no truth. Freud's critique is brief, powerful and remarkably prescient. Whatever is made of the postmodernist contentions they have captivated some people and given ease to some contemporary psychoanalysts.

Aner Govrin gives them a sympathetic ear.[25] The relational approach in psychoanalysis, he writes,

> posited that there are no absolute truths out there waiting to be discovered by clever human minds, but only meanings to be constructed by two persons functioning together in a cultural context … This view regards the idea of any observer having a God's-eye truth as an erroneous and passe positivist outlook. Relational therapists claim that *all* knowledge is relative and perspectival – dependent on the particular character and situation of the knower. Knowledge is therefore unavoidably constructed from a specific perspective, and is constructed within a social matrix in a social context.
>
> (Govrin 2016, 91; my italics)

Taken literally and generally, the claim imputed to the relational therapists is obviously false. I know as facts that I have never been to the moon and that men do not grow on trees. The knowledge is neither relative nor perspective-dependent. If a therapist doubts that the patient before him was born on some date and had a mother, then he ought to retrieve his shingle straightaway. The radical Pyrrhonism implied in the passage undermines the distinction between true and false assertion, which supervenes on *a way the world is*. Without the distinction, our institutions of law, contract, the teaching of history, science and carpentry collapse.

But perhaps the postmodernist claims are intended to apply only at the level of *theory*. Theories compete, are revised and discarded; paradigms of what constitutes knowledge change. That is true but does not show that no theories are, or can be, correct. The Earth revolves around the sun, not the other way round. The point need not be pressed. But perhaps, more realistically, and I believe this is what Govrin had in mind, the claims are intended to apply specifically to the domain of psychoanalysis where observation, theory and interpretation are indeed bedeviled by uncertainty and are often situation dependent. Still, we can manage to distinguish clear-cut cases of clinically relevant facts from theory-laden interpretation. In the course of an analysis it may become immensely important whether, for example, a patient as a child was actually raped. Of course, uncovering whether that is true or not may be difficult, but if it did happen then that is a fact, a historical fact like the battle of Waterloo, and likely to be critical to the course of analysis. The *fact* is not a matter of construction between two people; *uncovering* the fact, if it is a fact, may involve such constructions. I don't mean to imply that teasing out facts from constructions is easy, but some psychoanalysts have been so carried away by the obstacles to determining what is in another person's mind that they have to assume that there is nothing there, like the phenomenalists who think that trees cease existing when they are unobserved.

Overarching theories like Melanie Klein's or Kohut's are like any other theories, corrigible and revisable. Some theories answer to the facts better than others. But there is no principled reason to disbelieve that one day a relatively comprehensive clinical theory will answer to all or nearly all the facts garnered from a variety of sources: clinical, infant observation, neuroscience, anthropology and so forth. If there are principled reasons for skepticism, they have not been articulated by their would-be sponsors. Govrin writes that 'After some three decades during which postmodernism dominated the field and had a broad and profound influence on every aspect of western life, its ascendency has begun to wane' (2016, 139). I believe that this influence has been much exaggerated. Physicists, engineers, chemists and carpenters have continued their work of careful measurement and calculation undisturbed by anxieties over perspectivism. In the major centers of academic philosophy, where students cut their teeth on Protagorean relativism, postmodernist influence has been peripheral.[26] As best I can tell (I stand to be corrected), postmodernist influence has not extended to psychoanalysts working in an ego-psychological and object-relational framework, such as Otto Kernberg and his associates (Kernberg 2023), to neuro-psychoanalysis, psychodynamic neuroscience (Fotopoulou et al. 2012), the infant observers, and probably many other sectors of the community (Eagle 2022).

Not surprisingly, postmodernist conceptions have elated some of the religious. The tribunal of Reason is vanquished, and science and religion are on equal footing. As one postmodernist theologian typically expressed it, there is

> no view from nowhere or timeless ahistorical answer: there is no one right answer to most questions. There are many different and competing beliefs and practices and we should make every reasonable effort to accommodate them, to let many flowers bloom. Including the flower of religion … there is not a reason on earth (or in heaven) why many different religious narratives cannot all be true.
>
> (Caputo 2005, 63, 110)

Of course, many beliefs and narratives not only compete, they contradict. The willingness to entertain contradiction, paradox and the impossibility of truth is fatal to postmodernism and devastating for religion understood in any reasonably orthodox or traditional sense. Freud scorned the implicit intention to let religion in the back door by eliminating the test of truth, but he does not quite drive home its corrosiveness to traditional religion. The God who views the world from the perspective of eternity and omniscience, who has given His inerrant Word in Holy Books, who is the Truth and the Way, must be a fiction.

One might be forgiven for thinking that Freud exaggerated the conflict between science and religion as well as the intellectual privations and morbidities induced by religious teaching and institutions. If I may speak in the first person for a moment, I believe he got this exactly right. Even if the ferocious history of religious wars and depredations were put aside, we witness today declared Christian nations, Russia, the United States and others, dominated by Christian nationalists, scapegoating and persecuting outsiders, waging wars on weaker nations, and on science, medicine and the humanities.[27] Rational discourse has lost its grip on their politics. We live, as it is said, in a post-truth world. Where religious reactionaries have achieved political heft, in the Abrahamic, Hindu or Buddhist worlds, tolerance of religious, ethnic or sexual difference is under assault. As Freud said, on the matter of cruelty and intolerance the irreligious do better (Freud 1921c, 98). The world today is the world Freud in the 1920s thought was being left behind. It is ironic that when he was writing *The Future of an Illusion* the god *Logos* appeared to be ascendant. He expressed hope for the future. 'The primacy of the intellect lies, it is true, in a distant, distant future, but probably not an *infinitely* distant one' (1927c, 53). Its goals, 'the love of man and the decrease in human suffering', will be achieved gradually for a new generation of men.

> On the way to this distant goal … religious doctrines will have to be discarded … You know why: in the long run nothing can withstand reason and experience, and the contradiction which religion offers to both is all too palpable.
>
> (1927c, 54)

The final sentences of that work are appreciably muted. 'No, our science is no illusion. But an illusion it would be to suppose that what science cannot give us we can get elsewhere' (1927c, 56). Just a few years later, *Civilization and its Discontents* is somber. Freud thought that he was living at the beginning of an age of Reason and Science; the truth as it now appears is that he was living in parallel to a much larger world of latent religious inspiration that is now darkly reasserting itself.

Notes

1 Few academic philosophers today believe that the arguments Brentano presented are sound. Few, though there numbers are growing in the United States, believe that *any* arguments for God's existence are sound. Mackie 1982; Gale 1993; Martin 2007b; Oppy 2018 are good guides. The philosopher and psychoanalyst Jon Mills goes over the ground (and much else) in Mills 2017. 'Is there a God' is debated in contemporary perspective in Oppy and Pearce 2022.
2 The intellectual ferment of late 19th century and early 20th century Vienna has been well mined by historians and biographers. Cockett 2024, Chapters 1–4 gives a lively and informative account.
3 It does not follow that science does not deliver certainties, as David Black, for example, states in his introduction to a notable anthology (Black 2006a). Of course, it does: William Harvey discovered how the heart pumps blood. Nor does his glibly citing Kant's antinomies demonstrate that 'philosophy could not settle the questions of religion' and so should be left at that (2006a, 1).
4 See, e.g., Oppy 2018, Chapter 2.
5 I am using 'supernatural' synonymously with 'non-natural' although in some contexts there will be important differences; these need not be considered here.
6 Ernst Kris introduction to Freud 1954 [1887–1902] is still well worth reading as are several pertinent chapters of Solms 2015. Some philosophers see parallelism and dual aspect monism as entailing property dualism, and therefore as inconsistent with materialism. The issue remains contested. In a burgeoning literature, Hopkins 2012 and 2019 bring Freud's *Project* into the context of recent advances in the neuroscientific understanding of thought and phantasy. See also Pataki 2019.
7 See Parsons 2021 Chapter 6 for an extended discussion.
8 Argued, for example, in Symington 1998 and Parsons 2021.
9 Nearly everything Freud wrote about religion in the major works on culture (1912–1913, 1921c, 1927c, 1930a, 1933a, 1939a) as well as passing remarks in other significant works (e.g., 1907b, 1910c, 1918b) is of enduring interest and value.
10 Interest in how notions of *spirit* originated and their formative role in religion has revived in recent years and is now a central concern of cognitive anthropology. See, e.g., Barrett 2007; Guthrie 2007b; Lewis-Williams 2010; Whitehouse 2007. For critical discussion Pataki 2024, Chapter 3.
11 Freud believed at this time that an important difference between 'primitive' man and the 'civilized' is that the latter internalizes whereas the former projects. On the omnipotence of thought Pataki 2014, 69ff and the references to the classical literature there.
12 Religion 'comprises a system of wishful illusions together with disavowal of reality, such as we in an isolated form find nowhere else but

in amentia, in a state of blissful hallucinatory confusion'. But, he adds, 'these are only analogies, by the help of which we endeavour to understand a social phenomenon; the pathology of the individual does not supply us with a fully valid counterpart' (Freud 1927c, 43).

13 On wish-fulfilment Pataki 2014, 2019. The pioneering work of Richard Wollheim 1971, 1993 and Jim Hopkins 2012, 2019 must be mentioned. Joseph Sandler covered some of the same ground with his notion of 'actualization', e.g., Sandler 1989; Sandler and Sandler 1998.

14 In boys – it is nearly always the religious development of boys that Freud had in mind – the projections serve to relieve or sublimate the homosexual position and fear of castration. Freud doesn't discuss this issue at length in the main works on religion but attends to it in the case studies of Schreber (Freud 1911c), the Wolfman (Freud 1918b, esp. 114–117), and his study of a demonological neurosis (1923d). The young Wolfman playing the role of Christ to God the Father could 'drain off' his unconscious homosexuality and at the same time accommodate his intense masochism. Freud observes that although the threats of castration emanated from women, the phylogenetic factor was more influential and 'it was from his father whom in the end he came to fear castration' (1918b, 86). The fear of homosexuality and emasculation in monotheistic dispensations could not be more evident than it is today in the culture wars over gender identity and LGBTQ rights.

15 There is a heterogenous range of important work within a psychodynamic framework that the want of space precludes me from considering. I would mention Faber 2004; Ostow 2007; Merkur 2014; Mills 2017; and several papers by Rachel. B. Blass 2006, 2019.

16 A notable exception is described in Dodds, 1965, 43ff.

17 Horton 1997, 374–375; Brown 2018, 62 ff is a brilliant discussion.

18 The assumption is of course that monotheism and Buddhism are 'higher' religions than the polytheism of ancient Greece and Rome (and India). David Hume (1998 [1757]) thought that the polytheism was in better shape ontologically and morally than Christianity; as do I.

19 Jones 1957, Chapter X and Paul 2021, Chapter III for useful discussion. Freud liked to be in opposition, and Jones and subsequent commentators have created the impression that only Freud's obstinacy adhered him to Lamarckism. It was a surprise to learn of the intense debate in Vienna in the 1920s and 1930s on this question, with many leading biologists of the time, notably Paul Kammerer, on the Lamarckian side. The debate had political overtones. Nazi geneticists such as Fritz Lenz favored Darwinism which in their understanding suggested immutability of human types. Lamarckism allowed for rapid adaptation by the beneficial manipulation of the social environment, and so was favored by the Viennese socialists with whom Freud was in sympathy (Cockett 2024, Chapter 6).

20 Most readers of Freud conclude that spirits and gods derive from the totem, as Freud says explicitly in *Moses and Monotheism* (1939a, 83) and less explicitly in *Totem and Taboo* (1912–1913, 93). The view appears to be, as Paul expresses it that 'The totem animal, in the course of the evolution of civilization, became the basis for all subsequent supernatural beings, culminating in the omnipotent lone God of monotheism' (Paul 2021, 23). In fact, Freud's view is unresolved. In the *Wolfman* he tells us that 'I there (in *Totem and* Taboo) decided in favor of the view that God was not a development from the totem, but replaced it after arising independently from a root common to both ideas. The totem, I maintained, was the first father-surrogate, and the god was a later one' (1918b, 114). The relevant passages in *Totem and* Taboo (148–149) don't quite bear this out and he seems to want a bet each way. 'The answer might be that in the meantime the concept of God had emerged – from some unknown source – and had taken control of the whole of religious life; and that … the totem meal had been obliged to find a point of contact with the new system' (147). It is in any case difficult to square the totemic story with the asseverations in the opening chapter of *Future of an Illusion* concerning the birth of spirits. On the advent of spirits, Pataki 2024, Chapters 1 and 2.

21 See Paul 2021, 35ff.

22 Freud considered the legends of the Patriarchs to be tendentious and 'clumsy' narrative inventions (1939, 44–45).

23 It is often claimed that Freud hoped psychoanalysis would 'replace' religion (e.g., Parsons 2021; Meissner 1984). Freud's thought was that certain functions of religion, for example the cure of psychological maladies, imperfectly performed, would be better performed by psychoanalysis. The rest would fall by the wayside as science advances.

24 There are many versions of correspondence theories. Freud leaves open what specifically he had in mind. The philosophical literature on truth is vast and sophisticated but appears to be largely unknown in psychoanalysis. Good exceptions are by a philosopher turned psychoanalyst Hanly 2023, Caspi 2023 and Yadlin-Gadot 2023. Williams 2002 is a wide-ranging study by a major philosopher. *The Stanford Encyclopedia of Philosophy* under 'Truth' provides comprehensive and up to date treatment.

25 Govrin 2016, Chapters 2 and 4 where the relational approach to psychoanalysis is closely assimilated to postmodernist thought. How far, if at all, that assimilation is a theoretical or clinical *necessity* is a separate issue.

26 The French, of course, are another story, as are some literary critics and sociologists of science for whom postmodernism was philosophy-made-easy in five simple steps. Richard Rorty springs to mind as a significant exception though he is probably better classified as a late epigoni of American pragmatism.

27 As I write, I read that in Texas philosophy professors have been forbidden to teach Plato on the grounds that he challenges government proscriptions against gender identity and race related subjects.

Chapter 2

Ana-Maria Rizzuto and W. W. Meissner

Two orthodox critics and their criticism

The critique of Freud

The suggestion that Freud's aversion to religion arose from an uncompromising love of truth is likely to seem suspect to the religious and, for different reasons, to the psychoanalytically informed. It was inevitable that the instrument Freud created would be turned on him personally and onto the adequacy of his theoretical constructions. Broadly speaking, the internal criticism takes three forms. First, that Freud was not quite as irreligious (or, at least, 'unspiritual') as he made out. Second, that his views on religion were rooted in, and distorted by, the neurotic sectors of his personality. These two arguments are not necessarily *ad hominem* but are usually advanced to soften up Freud's avowal of atheism. But third, with considerably more substance, there are the observations and arguments that highlight the errors and limitations in Freud's understanding of psychic development as they bear on religion.

Ana-Maria Rizzuto and William Meissner are two gifted psychoanalysts who have written extensively about the intersection of religion and psychoanalysis. Devout Catholics, both, Meissner was an ordained Jesuit with a knowledge of biblical scholarship and some lines of philosophy unusual among psychoanalysts. Both are Freudians in the school of American ego-psychology, broadly influenced by British object-relations theory, Donald Winnicott especially. We shall say a few words about their positive contributions presently, but since both wrote extensively on Freud's

DOI: 10.4324/9781003508700-2

personal dispositions, suggesting that these weakened his theoretical positions, it is best to consider those arguments first. Moreover, their criticisms raise important questions within psychoanalytic theory that will recur at several junctions of our larger discussion. The first form of criticism is detailed by Meissner in his *Psychoanalysis and Religious Experience* (Meissner 1984) in a chapter titled 'Freud's Religion'. Meissner argues that Freud's attitude to religion or 'the spiritual' was, while unaccommodating, at least equivocal, as evidenced by his superstitiousness and preoccupation with the occult. According to Meissner, Freud was uncommonly superstitious. It must be said at once that it is easy to glance over a long life and from a high latitude accumulate instances of moods and follies. Poring over Freud's life, it is evident that he was superstitious: about death, travel and some numerological associations (Jones 1957, Chapter 14). My own assessment of the evidence is that Freud was about as superstitious as the average fellow, but perhaps my socializing with people who gamble and worry incessantly about death and travel biases the assessment. In any case, being superstitious hardly qualifies one for the mantle of religion. So, Meissner has to compound the imputation of superstitiousness with what he calls 'Freud's mystical tendency', that is, his interest in the occult. Putting them together, Meissner segues from Freud's superstitiousness (which is a trivial fact) to the alleged 'mystical tendencies' (the interest in the occult, which is a fact) to what he refers to as the 'religious aspects of Freud's personality' (Meissner 1984, 26f, 39ff, 41ff). This is a curious endpoint because it presupposes that being superstitious and interested in the occult implies religion. It is doubtful that is the conclusion Meissner intended.

Freud undoubtedly was interested in the occult. He went to some trouble tracking down mediums, holding seances in his home and experimenting with thought transference. Jung and Ferenczi, as is well known, dipped deeply into the occult, and it is obvious from Jones' account that Freud's characteristic astuteness deserted him when he was most intimately involved with them. Freud gave short shrift to most occult phenomena, poltergeists, revenants and so forth, but remained open to the possibility of thought transference or telepathy. The suggestion by Meissner and like-minded critics then is this: if Freud was sympathetic to the idea of occult processes, why not the spiritual, the religious or supernatural also? (Lev 2023, 15–16). The suggestion, however, misconceives Freud's interest in the occult. It lacks context. Freud's lifetime was a period of extraordinary scientific advance in which all phenomena, including the 'psychical' and the occult, were deemed admissible objects of scientific investigation. Many leading scientists and philosophers experimented with the occult. The physicist J. J. Thompson, William James, J. J. Putnam and C. D. Broad the distinguished Cambridge philosopher, to name a few, were active in psychical research (Broad 2011 [1962]). Freud was with them, although he declined several invitations to join the boards of august societies conducting this research. To one such, he wrote, incriminatingly according to his critics, that had he his life over he would have devoted it to psychical research (Meissner 1984, 38). It is well to recall (again) that people, even geniuses, have moods and whimsies. Freud's considered articles on the subject tell us that he saw his investigations in the light of the scientific *Weltanschauung* as 'an extension of the scientific – or, as our opponents say, the mechanistic mode of thought to the mental phenomena which are so hard to lay hold of' (1933a, 55). In a passage already cited, Freud notes that the majority of occultists are motivated to secure evidence for their religious faith; they are in fact 'convinced believers who are looking for confirmation', but analysts

> hope for the emergence of deeper-reaching natural laws, to which they are ready to submit. Analysts are at bottom incorrigible mechanists and materialists … they … embark on the investigation of occult phenomena only because they expect in that way finally to exclude the wishes of mankind from material reality.
>
> (Freud 1941d [1921], 178–179)

It is clear that Freud was inclined to explain thought transference by some as yet unknown *physical* substance serving as conduit, rather like a telephone connection (or Faraday fields of electromagnetism), and he thought that the recognition of unconscious processes made such telepathic communication more plausible. (We might surmise that his favorable reception of thought transference manifested a liminal awareness of communicative projective identification.) The leading motivation for his interest in the occult was scientific curiosity. Of course, emotional motives would have played a part, but it is a huge stretch to infer from Freud's occult interests to a metaphysical stance other than the naturalistic.

Freud's biographers have found abundant material ripe for psychoanalytic evaluation. The Catholic nanny who introduced the 2-year-old to Church services and religious ideas, and eventually disappointment, is alleged to have had a significant impact on Freud's attitudes to religion (though not by Ernest Jones, who thought the Church visits produced more theatrics than theology). Freud's unusual family dynamics, his disillusion with his father, the abandonments of his frequently withdrawn narcissistic mother, his prematurely enforced independence, his precocious reading of the Bible and alleged suppression of youthful religious propensities; such matters have been invoked to explain or to palliate Freud's hostility to religion. Gregory Zilboorg, Erich Fromm, W. W. Meissner, Neville Symington, Ana-Maria Rizzuto, Jeffrey Rubin and many others have made such connections, not unreasonably.[1] The attention to these matters is appropriate; the inferences from them are of variable merit. Rizzuto's *Why Freud Rejected God* (Rizzuto 1998) is probably the most scholarly psychodynamic case. Its title explains itself. It is impossible here to look into these connections in detail, but the premises supporting most of them require examination for their broader implications.

Meissner sets out the standard premise:

> It seems that Freud's religious views … reflect underlying and unresolved ambivalences and conflicts stemming from the earliest psychic strata. Behind the Freudian argument about religion stands Freud the man, and behind Freud the man, with his prejudices, beliefs and convictions, lurks the shadow of Freud the child. A basic psychoanalytic insight says that the nature and content of any thinker's or creative artist's work reflect essential aspects of the dynamic configurations and conflicts embedded in the individual's personality structure. Freud is no exception.
>
> (Meissner 1984, vii)

He concludes that 'Freud's rationalism and his agnostic belief were not free from conflict and clearly rested on powerful underlying motivations' (Meissner 1984, 55).

Meissner knows what the 'genetic fallacy' is and warns against it, but he is very much disposed to commit it anyway. It is evident that even if Freud's views about religion 'reflected' or, more precisely, were caused by dynamic and conflictual configurations that putative fact is irrelevant to whether the views are true or false. Whether Freud's atheism is true or not depends on whether there is a god or not of the kind whose existence Freud denies. What unconscious psychodynamic factors, if any, were involved is irrelevant to the truth of the matter.

But it is necessary to go further and probe the 'basic insight' to which Meissner refers. Many psychoanalysts believe, as Melanie Klein seems to have believed, that *all* mental processes involve unconscious object relationships. That may be true, or close to being true, of mental processes in patient and therapist in the course of treatment, but it is, of course, not true generally. Solving quadratic equations does not involve object relationships and generally does not involve unconscious (proximate) causal antecedents of any kind.[2] It may be true that much of what a person thinks and does, especially in creative work, has an unconscious *meaning* for that person and then, if communicated, perhaps for others. It is not true that everything a person thinks and does has dynamically unconscious (proximate) *causes.* Meissner's lazy word 'reflects' obscures the distinction. When an accountant is doing your tax return, you had better hope she is following the rules of accountancy and arithmetic, uninfluenced by unconscious motives. Much behavior is rule-following or constrained by 'the logic of the problem', or 'running into reality'. It is mostly so in mathematics and science, in carpet-laying and cooking. Whatever motives animated Einstein to try to reconcile special relativity with gravity, neither the motives nor their derivatives are to be found in the *content* of the General Theory of Relativity. The famous equations are a reflection (or perhaps only a refraction) of reality, not of human desire. Unconscious factors may, of course, intrude into most activities and create neurotic inhibitions and so forth, but that is not the rule.[3]

Speculative theories of religion of the kind that Freud created carry more emotional freight than mathematical theorems. Biases, conscious and unconscious, are conspicuously present in this work. But, to repeat, these factors are irrelevant to the truth value of the theories. Moreover, they are less significant than other factors that critics tend to ignore entirely. It is reprehensible that all the authors mentioned above neglect Freud's intellectual development after childhood, as if his education in science and humanities, his extended reading in the classics, history and philosophy, had no appreciable impact on him. We saw above that the opposite is the truth. To take one measure of this neglect, the name of Brucke does not appear in the indices of Meissner (1984), Symington (1998), Rizzuto (1998) or the anthology Black (2006a), nor in many other works of this ilk. Psychoanalysis has given full weight to the interpersonal and emotional factors that enter into belief formation. But humankind can, fortunately, be seized by rational argument and force of evidence. Some matters are demonstratable. The arguments for the existence of God with which Brentano probably tantalized the young Freud, for example, have been demonstrated to be unsound (Mackie 1982; Gale 1993; Martin 2007b). New arguments have come along. We know today, after two millennia of intense philosophical deliberation, that conceptions of immaterial spirits, psyches and souls face insuperable difficulties. *Logos* is indeed a mightier god than even Freud was willing to credit. It seems likely, then, that the *effective reasons* why Freud rejected theistic arguments was because he thought them bad arguments, not because he was conflicted, though, of course, he *was* conflicted; rejected religion and God (in Rizzuto's words) largely because of the incompatibility between religious belief and science, not because emotional factors blinkered him; criticized religion's intellectual and moral vices because he perceived them to be deplorable; and developed accounts of the origins of religion and religiosity that were reasonable, if ultimately unviable, constructions out of plausible anthropological and psychological materials, articulating at the same time some of his inner conflicts.

It goes without saying that these critics' explorations are partially motivated by the wish to paint Freud, and by implication all atheists, in pathological shades, just as they believe that Freud had pathologized religion. An interesting irony appears. Meissner and

Rizzuto accept the essential Freudian architecture for religiosity arising, in the earliest instances, in the cradle of the family: the earliest images of God are modeled on those of parents, and they accept that much religious observance is pathological. Meissner accepts the 'inherent validity' of the Freudian account (Meissner 1984, 68). 'In fact', he writes, 'we can safely say that the great mass of believers lend credence to Freud's formulations' (15). But both thinkers observe that Freud's architecture is incomplete, with glaring gaps at the foundations as well as its higher reaches. They are surely correct, and their own contributions rectify some of the defects. The irony is that their complaint that Freud failed to allow for the higher reaches of religious attainment beyond the oedipal constellations is much the same as their ignoring Freud's intellectual development beyond early adolescence. Meissner complains that in Freud's account there is 'no place for the more disciplined exercise of reason and intellect in the search for religious truth' (68). Freud's 'theological ignorance' precluded him from understanding the loftier and profound dimensions of 'mystical experience' (8). Meissner emphasizes religion's role in integrating and preserving the individual's sense of integrity and identity, which, when achieved, may be 'loosely called "spiritual"' (72). 'The religious enterprise is in many respects a quest, a striving within the ego to define an ultimate meaning, a personal significance, for oneself in the broader context of existence' (133). In the same key, Rizzuto writing about Freud's early essay on 'Obsessive Actions' (1907b) condemns Freud's 'ignorance of core aspects of religious experience … He says nothing about religion's efforts to understand the universe, to relate to a transcendent reality, to acknowledge human limitations and fragility while wondering about mysteries exceeding the powers of the intellect' (Rizzuto 1998, 159).

Rizzuto's protest is especially surprising.[4] On the face of it, it is difficult to think of a single plausible contribution that religion has made to the *understanding of the universe.* That would have something to do with space-time and quantum fields and so forth. It is hard to know what she is thinking of. It is curious that Rizzuto would expect Freud to expatiate on relations to a transcendent reality that he does not believe exists, or feel obliged to wonder about mysteries exceeding the powers of the intellect. Science and philosophy (by and large) represent piecemeal progress and the recognition of the limits of human understanding, of recognizing that the answer to many fundamental questions is that *we just don't know*, but might eventually. How different that is from the omnipotent thinking and dogmatic presumptions of religious thought.

In fact, both thinkers are committed to certain dogma from which their views necessarily evolve. Both believe that religious experience is epistemologically significant, profound and lofty. 'There is no area of human endeavor or existential involvement more profound, more far-reaching, more full of implication and significance than religious experience' (Meissner 1984, 6). But this understanding of religion as going deep is also highly parochial. It would surprise an Athenian of the 5th century BCE, a Viking warrior, or most Chinese people today; in fact, most of the globe's population today, for whom religion, except when it excites opportunities for group animosity, is rarely foremost. If we are to learn about religion and about human nature from its religious practices and beliefs, then we must subtend from the largest historical and cross-cultural arcs, beginning with the various forms of shamanism going back perhaps 20,000 years, attending especially to polytheistic systems which would confound much contemporary theorizing, and the much younger monotheisms. This seems obvious, so it is a little surprising to find (until one thinks about it) that for Meissner (and Rizzuto) the consequences of the anthropological and psychological research entailed by such a program would largely be beside the point. For them, neither the truth nor character of religion is contingent on empirical facts. As Meissner says, the psychology of religion can have nothing to say about the 'supra-human', the supernatural or divine aspects of religion and 'has no resources even to attempt to understand that loftier dimension' (1984, 6). The 'supra-human' refers, of course, to the transcendent being and to divine revelation. For both thinkers, the supernatural being of God and Christian Revelation is foundational. 'If one presupposes that there is no revelation and no revealing god, faith becomes totally meaningless and bizarre. But these presuppositions are themselves without convincing reality' (110).

Why should we believe that the presuppositions, the anti-theistic arguments and related considerations, are unconvincing? Broadly speaking, in the Catholic tradition there are three apologetical strategies. First, rational proofs of the existence of God, of the sort that Brentano introduced to Freud (probably Aquinas' 'Five Ways') and more recent theistic arguments, are affirmed to be valid; hence God exists, and there is reason to have faith in God's Revelation. Second, the deliverances of religious experience, the ecstasies and mystical encounters of the great mystics are said to be sources of knowledge and point to a transcendent reality. Third, the lives and spirituality of saints show, as in a glass darkly, the conformations of the divine.

Let's reserve for later discussion the supposed mystical and spiritual paths to knowledge and focus for the present on the first line of apologetics. It has to be acknowledged as an honest approach. In theistic religions everything turns on the truth of propositions about the gods. No-one, or nearly no-one, wants their religious beliefs to be based on falsehoods. And the best way to establish the truth of a proposition about gods is by evidence or metaphysical arguments, which psychoanalysis is neither in a position to provide nor to refute. So, Meissner completely detaches questions about the truth of theism from psychology and shifts them into philosophy or theology. But then, if psychoanalysis cannot finally contribute to determining the truth or otherwise of fundamental religious beliefs, what can it do that is relevant to the matter?

Well, of course, it can do a great deal, as we have already seen. In rough summary, Freud began the process of providing an epigenetic account of how religious concepts and beliefs are acquired, stressing as always the defensive and emotional aspects of the process. This account he saw as undermining, though not as refuting, religious belief, an important point which Meissner and Rizzuto tend to ignore. He showed that psychoanalysis can shine light on the role of religion in the processes of civilization and criticized its pernicious consequences for the individual and society. His many anthropological and historical speculations framed from the psychoanalytic point of view remain interesting, and in appreciable instances are still probably valid. Freud also gave some hints, but not many, concerning psychoanalytic treatment of individuals when religious thought is a special feature, as in some of the famous case histories. In a word, Freud mapped out the broad domain of intersection between religion and psychoanalysis, and since his time many features have been filled in by others.

Freud, however, almost entirely ignored the crucial role of the mother as the infant's first love object and nurturer. We saw one important reason for this exclusion in the area of religious formation – the theoretical need to fuse the paternal representation with the phylogenetic memory trace of the primal father. There were several other reasons, well known and of broader significance. Freud was also wont to exclude the possibility of significant religious development post-oedipally. He writes little about mystical experience, mystical doctrines, conversion, or those matters (whatever exactly they are) that Meissner describes as lofty and profound. Presumably, such matters provoked his skepticism. Meissner and Rizzuto, and several theorists we will consider presently, have been much less skeptical. They separately adopted Freud's epigenetic model for the development of religiosity, expanded and modified it to include the impact of pre-oedipal and post-oedipal experience. Rizzuto collated statistical and questionnaire data, using what Freud called 'American methods', and interpreted it through a psychoanalytic prism (Rizzuto 1979; McDargh 2017). Both of them focused on the emergence and evolution of the mental representations of God – images or concepts – and both emphasize the part that parents play initially in shaping these representations. (Rizzuto distinguishes between God images and God concepts, the latter associated with secondary process thinking, but that doesn't matter for the limited discussion here.) Unlike Freud, Rizzuto sees the relationship to God – or rather to the evolving God representation – in a benign light, indeed as potentially salvific. We cannot enter into details of Rizzuto's research, but having criticized premises of the attachment theory approach to the evolution of religiosity, something should be said about Rizzuto's position, which in several ways anticipated the later development.

Briefly then, Rizzuto concluded that most people in Western societies have conscious and unconscious representations of a being denoted by 'God' or some equivalent name. This is an unexciting finding. Children listen to talk, and in religious environments are exposed to rites centered around invisible objects and their representations. Soon they are taught how to relate to them, how to pray, genuflect, display the appropriate emotions and signs, and so forth. In the capacious sense of 'representation' that Rizzuto exploits, children form representations of real and unreal objects, events, fictions and possibilities; these become objects of thought. Rizzuto insists that God representations are not exclusively based on the father imago; they undergo evolution under the influence of mothers crucially, of other significant persons, cultural influences and indeed a person's own rational reflections. She does not include *direct* experience of God and does not err by drawing ontological conclusions from the fact that people have God representations. But by failing at critical points to distinguish between representations and the object represented, and between *kinds* of representation, she lands in a muddle. She writes: 'If one is willing to accept that a mature relationship with one's parents is possible, then a mature relationship with the God representation should also be possible' (Rizzuto 1979, 52; McDargh 2017, 17). Not to put too fine a point on it, there are differences between relating to a flesh and blood parent and to a mental representation (or, say, icon) of a parent; and between relating to a flesh and blood parent and the representation of an incorporeal being. Even if the conflation Rizzuto canvasses 'should be possible', it remains obscure on her account how it occurs. Oral Roberts, the influential Pentecostal preacher, tells how in his childhood his parents prayed to Christ in such a conversational manner that 'I actually thought that Christ lived in our house, was a member of the family' (Fitzgerald 2018, 211). Roberts presumably had an unusually robust representation of Christ, but it is unlikely to have been as laden with meaning as the representation of his mother, and he could scarcely have mistaken one for the other. The formation of mother images is crucially dependent on vicissitudes of attachment involving physical and emotional interaction, reliable presence, mirroring, and so forth. Incorporeal objects like God don't meet the job description. On the face of it, her account confronts the same difficulties that attachment theorists have in explaining how intense attachment to incorporeal objects is possible. Freud's solution to the problem was that the paternal representation (or internal object) is projected into the (representation of) God, so that unconsciously they are experienced as one and the same. Rizzuto can go along with that, but only up to a point. She argues that as the God image undergoes modification in the course of normal development it can become untethered from its original core in the parental identification. But if so, then it becomes difficult to explain how the intense relationship to the God image – to God – can persist. The dynamics of Freud's solution, with all its explanatory gains, is not open to her on pain of acknowledging the essentially infantile character of the relationship. She wants, to use Freudian jargon, to retain intense emotional cathexis directed onto the God representation without fixation to the parental imago. That appears to be problematic.

Enter Donald Winnicott: illusion and muddle

Rizzuto, Meissner and others staked a lot on Winnicott's notion of the transitional object and his claim that cultural experience, including religious experience, occurs in a transitional or potential space, a 'third' area of experience. The mother allows, Winnicott wrote,

> the infant the illusion that what the infant creates really exists. This intermediate area of experience, unchallenged in respect of its belonging to inner or external (shared) reality, constitutes the greater part of the infant's experience, and throughout life is retained in the intense experiencing that belongs to the arts and to religion.
>
> (Winnicott 1974 [1971], 16)

Taken to apply to all artistic and religious experience, the claim, although repeated frequently and taken on faith, is patently false. Winnicott probably had in mind something like Ernst Kris' notion of the 'aesthetic illusion' in which, even in adult experience, imagination and reality mingle, with a loss of reality testing as in engrossment in the theater.[5] Perhaps he was thinking of his own experience in the solemnity of the cathedral, the regressive pull of the cave and womb.[6] The details need not concern us; we know that something like 'illusional' experiences in art and religious devotion occur, if only sporadically. However, the spatial metaphors conceptually reduce and distort the enormous *variety* of these experiences. The theater, movies, novels and visits to sacred places can leave us cold, but are cultural encounters nonetheless; folk dancing, communal beer-drinking, building pyramids and cathedrals, marriages and attending funerals may also be religious events. There is no need to question Winnicott's insights into the infant's relation to transitional objects, or indeed whether metaphorical constructions like 'potential space' or 'third area of experience' make any sense. One might indeed wonder where the second 'area of experience' is supposed to occur. However, we have good reason to be cautious of supposing that such metaphors are useful in illuminating cultural and, specifically, religious experience.

Rizzuto is impressed by the similarity between the infant's construction of transitional objects and the construction of the God image from the infant's inner world and the externally given object. She is persuaded by Winnicott's claim that transitional experience perdures through the life span; as she herself argues that God images perdure and are modified over the life span. So, she concludes that '*psychologically* God is a transitional object' (Rizzuto 1979, 177). The force of the qualification 'psychologically' is not entirely clear. Others who follow Rizzuto assert without qualification that God *is* a transitional object, *simpliciter*, a claim that is obviously false, for then there would be as many gods as individuals having transitional objects.[7] The import seems to be, as best I can understand it, that God is neither entirely inner nor entirely outer. God is an illusion, as 'illusion' is understood in the Winnicottian scheme of things. That, of course, is not great news for the traditional religious believer for whom God preceded us, created the world, and has powers we can't imagine. Meissner works hard to show that many aspects of religious belief and practice – faith, prayer, God representations – are transitional or illusional in the Winnicottian sense (Meissner 1984, Chapter 7). He approves of Rizzuto's conclusion that:

> Like other transitional objects, the experience of God or the God representation is neither a hallucination nor is it totally beyond the reach of subjectivity; rather it is located, in Winnicott's terms, 'outside, inside, at the border' (Winnicott (1974) [1971], 2). Unlike the teddy bear or the blanket, God is created out of representational derivatives that stem particularly from the child's experience of primary objects.
>
> (Meissner 1984, 179)

Notice the systematic confusion between God and God's representation. The experience of God, whatever exactly that is (perhaps a mystical encounter), is not the same as having a God representation; and the entity God, whatever exactly God is, is not created out of representational derivatives. Of course, people will have their own images of God constructed, perhaps, along the lines of transitional objects. But those images cannot *be* God on pain of multiplication of gods. This muddle derives, quite possibly, from conferring on the perspective of the infant in its transitional experience profound ontological significance. There is a vast difference between the way things seem to the infant – who we do not challenge because it would be pointless to do so – and the way things are. From this trickle of confusion, a vast river has emerged.

Freud defined 'illusion' prescriptively as *belief* engendered by wishes. He condemned illusions when they were false *and* sought to displace reality. Art, unlike religious belief, causes no offense because, though illusory, it does not seek to displace reality. Winnicott's notion of the illusional is entirely different from Freud's. In his hands, illusion acquires a kind of pseudo-reality forged of creative imagination and physical object. Foregoing this difference, Meissner and Rizzuto launch factitious critiques of Freud's position. Meissner writes glibly:

> If Freud wishes to rule out illusion and to destroy it, Winnicott wishes to foster it and increase man's capacity for creatively experiencing it. Winnicott sees that illusion is an important part of human experience precisely because it is not by bread alone

> that man lives … Winnicott's notion of psychic health is not the separation of the real and the wishful, as Freud might have had it, but rather their constant intermingling and exchange.
>
> (Meissner 1984, 177)

In ordinary usage, as well as in Freud's, *most* illusions – optical illusions, vain hopes and so forth – are indeed false or misleading. Winnicott would have caused far less confusion had he chosen other words from the English lexicon, 'creative imagination', perhaps. For without the distinction it appears that those like Meissner and Rizzuto who follow him down this track are prescribing the utility – the necessity? – of false beliefs, deception and self-deception in the service of creative life. This raises deep moral questions about the connections between seeking truth and intellectual self-respect and integrity.[8] But sidestepping truth may be the very point. It is not news that false beliefs, illusions, distorted self-conceptions can sustain and even improve 'psychic health' in the medical understanding of this notion. *Hope*, the ancient Greeks believed, was the worst of the vices, but it has sustained many a soul at the edge of hell since then. Possessing benign, loving God representations (in Rizzuto's sense) can help individuals (and their counselors and therapists) in negotiating the trials of life, just as cruel or envious representations may exacerbate them. God representations have their uses and liabilities. John McDargh quotes from William James (quoting a colleague) a passage which he says gives deeper resonance to Rizzuto's work:

> *God is not known, he is not understood; he is used* … If he proves himself useful, the religious consciousness asks for no more than that. Does God really exist? How does he exist? What is he? Are so many irrelevant questions. Not God, but life, more life, a larger, richer, more satisfying life, is, in the last analysis, the end of religion.
>
> (McDargh 2017, 30)

William James notoriously confused the truth of a proposition with its utility or value. It follows from this conflation that once we have utility – health, life, coping with despair – truth as an independent value is rendered superfluous. As Rizzuto says:

> Asking a mature, functional individual to renounce his God would be like asking Freud to renounce his own creation, psychoanalysis, and the 'illusory' promise of what scientific knowledge can do. This is, in fact, the point. Men cannot be men without illusions. The type of illusion we select – science, religion, or something else – reveals our personal history and the transitional space each of us has created between his objects and himself to find 'a resting place' to live in.
>
> (Rizzuto 1979, 209)

According to Rizzuto we can choose our illusion, whether it be 'science, religion, or something else'. Evidence, reason, truth, and the serious epistemological thought of the ages are irrelevant to the determination of our beliefs. The choice reveals – is determined by? – personal history and the transitional spaces we have created. There is no need for further comment. Rizzuto's line of thought leads to a sad, intellectually derelict 'resting place'.[9]

Freud's interlocutor in *The Future of an Illusion* accused him of replacing one illusion with another, the belief in transcendence with the illusion of humanity worshipping science, psychoanalysis in the vanguard, marching bravely forward without the brace of supernatural belief. Freud admitted the possibility of illusion, but with a critical proviso: 'my illusions are not, like religious ones, incapable of correction', he wrote. 'They have not the character of a delusion. If experience should show … that we have been mistaken, we will give up our expectations' (1927c, 53). In valorizing the primacy of the intellect and of science he was enjoining realism both about humanity and the prospect of exploring the universe outside it. That realism reflects love of truth, which is love of the world, of living with intellectual self-respect in a place where the intelligence strives to be free of illusion. Rizzuto suggested, at rather great length, that Freud's depreciation of illusion, his insistence on stoically confronting a stark world full of adversity, reflects the premature independence forced upon the young Freud as a 'parentified' child (Rizzuto 1998, 209ff). Something like that may well be true. Freud's insistence on living without the crutch of *wishful illusion*, on bending only to necessity, may originate from an upbringing in which independence was prematurely thrust upon him. But then it is an open question whether that experience obscured reality or allowed Freud a much clearer view and appreciation of it.

Notes

1 On still earlier critiques see Jones 1957. Parsons 2021, 35ff sums up several of the later ones.
2 I say 'proximate' because there may be developmental paths to such causes.
3 Heinz Hartmann and others observed that some ego-functions were autonomous from birth and others became autonomous in the course of development forming conflict-free spheres of the ego, primary and secondary (Hartmann 1958 [1939], 1964). Freud had earlier written of independent ego-interests and of the ego and superego acquiring independent sources of energy through neutralization of instinctual energies. Developing these distinctions, Hartmann and other ego-psychologists employed a number of energic conceptions, largely ignored since the severe critiques of the 1970s, although Hartmann had in fact good principled reasons for using them, set out in a number of early papers (Hartmann 1964). These were the best materials at hand, as he thought, to construct psychoanalysis as a causal science. Were Hartmann alive today he would probably be employing Karl Friston's free energy concepts (Hopkins 2019). It is unfortunate that the conceptions of ego autonomy he described are largely neglected in contemporary theorizing. However, see Eagle 2022. Hartmann frequently complained that psychoanalysis does not have a theory of action – of intention, choice, decision, intentional action and the cluster of concepts around them that are necessary for elucidating any notion of ego autonomy. It still has not. There is a rich literature on action theory in contemporary philosophy from which psychoanalysis could hugely profit. Davidson 1980 contains some of the seminal papers.
4 Perhaps it is because of failure to imagine an upbringing less saturated with God-talk than her own. Thus, she writes of the impact on the 2-year-old Freud of the departure of his Catholic nanny: 'Sigmund was left bereft of supports – nurse, church and God' (Rizzuto 1998, 242). A most improbable scenario and a baffling statement.
5 Kris 1952, 39ff. Kris relates the story of the yokel who attends Shakespeare's *Julius Caeser* for the first time. At the crucial moment he stands and shouts 'Watch out, they're armed!' Pataki 2014, Chapter 2 discusses attention and engrossment in some detail.

6 Lewis-Williams 2010 provides a most interesting discussion of the hallucinogenic effects of parietal art in Palaeolithic caves and the similarities in outlay of sacred caves and later constructions such as cathedrals. Biographers have noted Winnicott's lingering religiosity although he criticized religions for being closed dogmatic systems that thwarted individual creativity. In particular, he deprecated 'moral' education not built on the child's inherent morality (Dobbs 2007, 117). Clare Winnicott said that D. W. was never 'anti-religion' and 'was only too thankful if anybody could believe anything' (Dobbs 2007, 118). D. W. was, it is to be hoped, referring to the *capacity* 'to believe in', to have basic trust, that he discusses in 'Morals and Education' in his book (Winnicott, 1965).

7 Leroy Howe quoted in McDargh 2017, 24, 37–38; cf. Meissner below.

8 Nietzsche raised these issues in acute form. 'Truth has to be fought for every step of the way, almost everything else dear to our hearts, on which our love and trust in life depend, has had to be sacrificed to it. Greatness of soul is needed for it, the service of truth is the hardest service'. With 'the will to truth', he writes, 'I will not deceive, not even myself … *with that we stand on moral ground*' (quoted in Williams 2002, 13).

9 Rizzuto argues that the 'psychic conditions' for religious belief and unbelief are on a par epistemologically, being dependent on developmental paths in early life. Freud was deprived of the conditions for belief that most people acquire and would have made him a believer (Rizzuto 1998, Chapter 12). There are many insuperable problems with this kind of internalism and they have been extensively exposed in the philosophical literature.

Chapter 3

Toward the abyss

Erich Fromm

Background

Some of Freud's immediate followers wrote about religion, at length and well. Theodore Reik, Ernest Jones, Karl Abraham, Geza Roheim, to mention only outstanding figures, extended Freud's observations on the symbolic character of religious dogmas and rituals and shared his atheism. Interestingly, Abraham published an early paper on Akhenaten's religion that Freud appears to have forgotten. Leaving Jung aside, the main critical voice at this time was Oskar Pfister, but for all of Freud's affection and respect for Pfister he did not take the criticisms seriously. Pfister's rhapsodic declamations were hardly likely to impress someone who knew the history of Western civilization far better than Pfister did.

> Religion is the sun that gave rise to the most splendid flowering of art and the richest harvest of moral convictions. Every great and powerful work of art is a prayer and a sacrifice before the throne of God … And we also see religion as the main foundation of morality.
>
> (Pfister, quoted in Meissner 1984, 98)

These are Sunday-school conceptions, and Freud thought them little more than flowery poetry.

In 1950, Erich Fromm, who was by then a somewhat unorthodox psychoanalyst, published a short book, *Psychoanalysis and Religion*, which had an influence far beyond its merits. It may be

DOI: 10.4324/9781003508700-3

taken as marking an early turning point in the psychoanalytic understanding of religion. Its impact on the wider population of psychoanalysts was perhaps not pronounced, but in the decades that followed notable analysts published work sharply at variance with the Freudian line. From our perspective this is the point at which psychoanalytic writing on religion begins its sharp decline: it detaches itself from anthropology and the biological sciences, from rigorous thought, epistemological reserve and serious philosophical debate about religion. In some quarters there follows a lurch into mysticism and vague, unarticulated spirituality.

Fromm had an orthodox Jewish background, but he seems to have separated himself from religious orthodoxy by his mid-20s and became an unorthodox Marxist. In his first major work, *The Dogma of Christ* (Fromm 2004 [1963]), he attempted to reconcile Freud and Marx by demonstrating in the case of early Christianity the reciprocal influences of psychological dispositions and social and economic conditions. He achieved this with very considerable success. He grew close to a group of American psychoanalysts – Karen Horney, Erik Erikson and others – who were also moving in a more sociologically orientated direction, at some variance with the greater emphasis on the inner world among the ego-psychologists and British object relations theorists. Although he renounced religious belief as understood traditionally, Fromm retained deep respect for the moral content of the Bible, especially for the Jewish prophets and their concern for social justice, as he interpreted them. This influenced not only the theoretical content of his writing but also, unfortunately, the grating prophetic tone of it: its repetitious exhortations to 'Man' about what he must and mustn't do, often about matters of which he had as little understanding as did the prophets. Three other factors were even more formative than his religious learning. The shattering events of the Second World War and the depredations of Stalin's ruthless dictatorship linked the pathology of the dictator with the psychological transformations undergone by people living in authoritarian dispensations. Fromm saw that authoritarian rule activates sadomasochistic dynamics conducive to converting people into unthinking parts of an unthinking machine. He acutely detected traces of authoritarianism in the Abrahamic religions. He was one of the first to see that the commodity capitalism sweeping the world after the war, although it produced great material wealth, led to the commodification of persons, the imposition of sadomasochistic postures reflecting authoritarian structures, and spiritual and, as he believed, religious hollowing out. Finally, in the decades after the war Buddhism, Zen Buddhism especially, was being introduced to the American public. Here appeared a religion, possibly atheistic, apparently peaceful or irenic (Japanese Buddhist militancy during the war being forgotten), conforming with the aims of psychoanalysis in mitigating suffering, achieving insight and finding inner peace. Fromm liked what he saw of it (Fromm and Suzuki 1993 [1960]). These various influences eventually led him to conflate religion, morality and a rarefied mysticism. He conducted one of those 'rearguard actions' that Freud warned about, stretching the meaning of words until nothing is left of the original sense, and 'religion' becomes the name of some amorphous principle. On the basis of a few superficial indications, he sought to detach religion from its historical and conceptual moorings and thereby effectively changed the subject. He got drunk on apple juice.

Definition of religion

From this point on there will be recurrent question marks over definitions of religion, so here is the place to introduce a serious one. It will not do to manufacture definitions at convenience. The following rather complex definition is the best I know:

> Religions are passionate, communal displays, of costly commitments to the satisfaction of non-natural causal beings – e.g., gods and/or ancestor spirits – and/or the overcoming of non-natural causal regulative structures – e.g., cycles of reincarnation, reward and punishment – resulting from:

1 widespread belief in non-natural causal agents and/or non-natural regulative structures;
2 hard to fake public expressions of costly material commitments – offerings and/or sacrifices of goods, property, time, and/ or life – to the satisfaction of those non-natural causal agents

and/or the overcoming of, or escape from, those non-natural causal regulative structures;

3 mastering of people's existential anxieties – death, deception, disease, catastrophe … by those costly commitments to the satisfaction of those non-natural causal agents and/or the overcoming of, or escape from, non-natural causal regulative structures; and

4 ritualized, rhythmic, sensory co-ordination of (1), (2) and (3) in communion, congregation, intimate fellowship or the like.[1]

The definition captures most religions acknowledged intuitively, those that recognize gods as well as those that recognize only lesser spirits or supernatural processes such as reincarnation. It excludes would-be religions such as Scientology, assuming its religious objects are natural entities (extra-terrestrial beings). It excludes political ideologies such as Nazism or Communism because commitment to spiritual beings, such as are intrinsic to the ideology, is lacking. It emphasizes ritual and sacrifice, but the main thread running through the definition is *belief in spirits or supernatural agents and processes.* Edward B. Tylor, we saw above, defined religion as belief in spiritual beings, and contemporary cognitive anthropology of religion and evolutionary psychology place the notion at the center of their studies of religion: there is substantial agreement among researchers that belief, or at least the disposition to believe, in spirits (including gods) is a necessary feature of all, or nearly all, religions.[2] Naturalistic forms of pantheism and panentheism are excluded. Borderline cases, Jainism and austere forms of Buddhism such as Theravada, are atheistic in principle and do count intuitively as religions. However, although Buddhism has in places glossed the older folk religions, the mass of believers have not surrendered their supernatural beliefs. There are probably more Buddhist atheists in California than Tibet. Belief in supernatural agencies and processes, as diverse as these may be, is inseparable from religion. It has been so since humans in the Late Paleolithic period pressed their palms onto the walls of shelters seeking contact with the spirits inhabiting them. Where belief in the supernatural is absent, it is more apt to speak of philosophies, moral reflection or hankerings for ecstatic or anomalous experiences. Today, the concept of the spiritual is often detached from the context that gave it sense and has become an honorific title. A person who is 'deep', loves art and the splendor of the natural world, is 'open to experience' or drawn to meditation, mystical experiences and self-exploration is likely to consider themselves spiritual, and, very likely, as religious.

Fromm made a distinction between 'authoritarian' and 'humanist' religion that initiated an influential pattern. James W. Jones decades later makes the same distinction; the famous psychologist Gordon Allport distinguished between immature and mature forms of religion; Neville Symington between primitive and mature religion; W. W. Meissner between neurotic and mature religion; and the psychoanalyst Paul W. Pruyser distinguished between neurotic or sick and healthy religion. These writers have a friendly disposition toward religion but concede contingent pathological flaws. So, they prescind from it, by fiat, what they don't like and defend the more congenial aspects. Those aspects are usually what philosophers and most ordinary people call ethics or morality, or reflection on these things, moral philosophy. The point of their exercises is, of course, to preserve some appealing content for religion, after most of what is typical of it has been cut away. The supernatural, the dogmatic, the sacrificial, the oblatory, the institutional, even the salvific elements are cast aside. What is left, however, misrepresents the religious enterprise as it has been in the past and as it is still understood by the vast majority of religious adherents.

Fromm says that by religion he understands 'any system of thought and action shared by a group which gives the individual a frame of orientation and an object of devotion' (Fromm 1978 [1950], 21). That definition is too inclusive to be useful. In my country, football and cricket satisfy the definition. Fromm then asserts that the need for a system of orientation is the most powerful need intrinsic to man. It follows from the conjunction of his definition and this supposedly powerful need that 'there is no-one without a religious need'. That seems obviously false, but Fromm's conjunction had opened the gates wide. Religious needs, he says, can be satisfied in the worship of animals, trees, idols, gods, gold, diabolical leaders and so forth. Now the conclusion is easy:

everyone is religious: the question is, '*not religion or not* but *which kind of religion*, whether it is one furthering man's development, the unfolding of his specifically human powers, or one paralyzing him' (Fromm 1978 [1950], 26). Fromm thinks that traditional religion has too often betrayed its stated ideals of love and humility in everyday life. So he winnows it, and makes his principal distinction 'which cuts across nontheistic and theistic religions: that between *authoritarian* and *humanistic* religions' (34). The essential element in the former is surrender to a power transcending man; obedience is its main virtue. Authoritarian religions paralyze, like neuroses, in that they defeat 'the fundamental aims of human existence, independence and the ability to be productive, to love, and to think' (28). Its 'spirit is one of submission to power and lack of love and of respect for the individual' (63). Calvinism is his chief theistic target and submission to the Führer is the main secular example of authoritarian religion.

Humanistic religion is utterly different. It is expounded by Fromm in a series of salutary imperatives, the intelligible parts of which may be abridged as follows. In humanistic religion 'Man' must develop his power of reason to understand himself and his fellow man; he must recognize the truth; must develop his powers of love for others as well as himself; must have principles and norms to guide him. Humanistic religion involves the experience of 'oneness with All' as the world is grasped with thought and love. In it, God is a symbol of Man's own powers, not a symbol of force and domination over him. The examples of humanistic religion Fromm provides are early Buddhism, Taoism, the teachings of Isaiah, Jesus, Socrates, Spinoza, all of which are 'essentially the same' in 'striving for love, truth and justice'; also included are certain mystical trends in the Jewish and Christian religions, the religion of Reason and the French Revolution. Fromm knew a good konditorei when he saw one. Of these, the best example, Fromm opines, is early Buddhism, for the Buddha 'recognizes the truth about human existence' (37–38). In searching for the humanitarian streak in Biblical tradition, Fromm relates a rabbinical tale of how God wanted Man to 'become his own master, capable and resolved to make his decisions by himself according to rational, democratic methods'. By this point, one wonders where

Fromm's critical sense is, whether he is capable of any discriminations at all. When he tells us that man will only attain the full capacity for objectivity and reason when 'loyalty to the human race and to its ideals is considered the prime loyalty that exists' (60) one wonders where his feet are. It is glib stuff, and its vacant moralism and innocence is embarrassing. What *are* these norms and principles that 'must' guide man, and what is *the* truth of human existence? Are Socrates, Jesus, Spinoza and Robespierre really on the same level? The only way of making sense of this is to realize that Fromm has altogether left the subject of religion behind. The amorphous thing he calls 'humanistic religion' is a well-meaning ethics of broadly humane, liberal, democratic ideals naively and haphazardly stacked together. Commendable ideals, but hardly definitive of any plausible understanding of religion.

Some of Fromm's observations on authoritarian aspects of religions are insightful. He notices a kind of projection or evacuation in which Man, 'already feeling small', idealizes God and impoverishes himself still further. Losing his best parts in this process, he becomes alienated from himself and, being left with the worst parts, feels himself a sinner. 'The more perfect God becomes, the more imperfect becomes man' (50). He 'begs God to return to him some of what was originally his own'. Both socio-economic and psychological forces drive this process. The latter comprise unconscious desires to be weak and powerless, to escape from freedom and responsibility. And Fromm also sees the sadistic obverse of the authoritarian character structure, its tendency to 'rule and dominate' (54). The sado-masochistic trends in the obsessional character that Fromm recognized – and here he is close to the seminal *Authoritarian Personality* of Theodor Adorno et al. (1950) – in Fascist authoritarianism also sheds a good deal of light on the dynamics of large religious institutions, evangelical movements and, of course, contemporary political dispensations. In this early work Fromm appears not to have discerned how the narcissistic idealization of, and identification with, the authoritarian leader serves to share in his grandiosity and desire to crush enemies, though the omission is remedied in later work (Fromm 1973). This aspect was already noticed by Freud (1921c) and has been much elaborated by many psychoanalysts in subsequent decades.

Fromm was one of the early critics of the ego-psychology of his time, whose therapeutic aim he misunderstood as being little more than social adjustment. Whether the ego-psychologists who, often by way of the therapeutic alliance, sought principally to strengthen the ego, enhance its capacities for rational judgment and moderate the superegos of their patients, were seeking nothing more than social adjustment is certainly moot. In any case, Fromm thought that the unalloyed therapeutic aim of social adjustment was based on a mistaken assumption of social relativism and ignored 'universal human norms' or the 'immutable laws inherent in human nature'. If the analyst does have such norms in mind, so Fromm claimed, then she is properly viewed as a physician of the soul whose aim is not the patient's social adjustment but the 'optimal development of a person's potentialities and the realization of his individuality' as these are prescribed by the universal norms (Fromm 1978 [1950], 74). And so, if religion is construed humanistically, as comprising the essentially curative aims common to all the great religious teachers, then psychoanalysis as a 'cure of the soul has very definitely a religious function' (76). That brave claim has been repeated many times since, and we shall consider it in more detail below.

Morality 101

What *are* the immutable laws that 'must' guide 'Man' and the physician of the soul to lead the patient to the optimal development of his potentialities and individuality? We are not told much. There is an interesting discussion of incest understood broadly as inability to separate from mother, clearly an impediment to independence and individuation, and so to freedom, as Fromm understands it. The drive to independence (separation and individuation) looks like a candidate for being an inherent human universal sustaining a moral norm. But Fromm does not elaborate or face the well-known difficulties of deriving normative (evaluative) propositions from factual ones. Instead, he repeats platitudes about the aims of life: independence, integrity, justice, and the ability to love truth and others, and so forth. No-one would wish to denigrate such virtues. At least in the Western tradition, apart from a few outliers like Callicles or Nietzsche, most people would agree that such things are good. It is much, much harder, as the entire history of Western thought shows, to get agreement on what these things *are*. To cite the prophets endorsing justice and righteousness without knowing what they *meant* by these things, as Fromm does, is an empty device. One suspects that they meant something quite other than what the Marxist Fromm had in mind. At the roots of Western moral philosophy Socrates gadded fellow citizens with questions such as What is piety? What is justice? What is courage? What is virtue (excellence)? What is knowledge? Socrates did not provide answers.[3] The questions are still there, much discussed in the academy and the marketplace, but Fromm gives no indication that he is aware of them. Yet without answers the physician of the soul is in a rather awkward position.

Freud thought that Jesus' injunction to love thy neighbor as thyself was neither realistic nor morally justifiable. Undiscriminating in its objects, the injunction diminishes the value of love for one's intimate circle. Fromm insists that the injunction is 'the most important norm of living in that its violation is the basic cause of unhappiness and mental illness' (87). Fromm misinterprets the injunction that Freud declines to approve. His interpretation is not that every human should be loved equally (as oneself), but that the *capacity* to love someone apart from oneself is critical to health. Freud had stated as much. That proposition is likely to be true, but Fromm draws from it a *non sequitur*: all neurotic symptoms are rooted in the inability to love, and analytic therapy is 'essentially an attempt to help the patient gain or regain his capacity for love' (87). This is an exaggeration, of course, but an anticipation of issues that are soon to loom very large in psychoanalysis. Fromm suggests a connection between the recession of love and the marketing orientation of contemporary society, but fails to clarify precisely, or even roughly, what that connection is.

Having detached his conception of religion from its traditional metaphysical, ritualistic and institutional moorings, Fromm is eventually compelled to ask how humanistic religion is to be distinguished from the realm of the ethical. His answer foreshadows the dismaying trend that was soon to emerge in some psychoanalytic quarters. The distinction between the ethical and humanistic religion lies in the *religious experiences* which are such that only those who experience them can understand (Fromm 1978 [1950], 94), a requirement that certainly limits the field of prospective critics. These experiences subsist in part on a set of attitudes: of wonderment, marveling at the world, being puzzled by existence, not taking existence for granted but feeling it as a problem which has as yet no answers. Of course, this agnosticism about the 'riddle of the world', in Wittgenstein's phrase, if not the inclination to marvel at it, would astound a devout Christian, Jew or Muslim for whom the answers have been revealed in Holy Scriptures. The attitudes of puzzlement would seem more characteristic of baffled atheists than the devout religious. But Fromm is not concerned with the religion of the legions, which is basically authoritarian in his terms, or with trivial distinctions between atheists and the devout. For him, 'religious' is an honorific term signifying a set of virtues and attitudes that he favors.

Another important element of humanistic religious experience is the attitude of *oneness with one's fellow man, with all life and with 'the All'*, that is to say, various states described by mystics of several religious traditions. With fellow-feeling and compassion extended to all living things, most mature adults have some acquaintance. What 'the All' could be is not made clear. Fromm explains that the path to 'the All' (as best I can follow it) runs through a mystical process which consists in the breaking down of ego structures and getting in touch with unconscious aspects of the self – not the unconscious of Freud or Jung, however, which Fromm says are distortions. He means the excluded part of the ego which contains the 'highest and the lowest', the best and the worst. This unconscious must not be approached as if it were a

> God whom we must worship or a dragon we must slay, but in humility, with a profound sense of humor … When we get in touch with this dissociated part, we retain the individuation of ego structure but we experience this unique and individualized ego as only one of the infinite versions of life …
>
> (Fromm 1978 [1950], 97)

These assertions, some blowing in from the East, others from late antiquity, are, of course, problematic, but since several aspects of mysticism will be discussed directly, we can leave Fromm at this point for another psychoanalyst of kindred spirit.

Notes

1 A slightly abridged version of Scott Atran's (2002) definition modified in Oppy 2018, 31. See also Martin 2007a. The definition is imperfect. Some religions do not involve passionate or costly displays. There is also a reasonable question about whether primitive fetishism involving worship of animals in the absence of a conception of *spirit* (if indeed there was such a thing) should count as religion.
2 Guthrie 2007; Barrett 2007; Whitehouse 2007; Bering 2011; Dunbar 2022.
3 In Plato's early 'Socratic dialogues'. In later dialogues, though still with Socrates as protagonist, Plato develops tentative answers to some of these questions and the metaphysics of the theory of Forms, something that would have been alien to Socrates.

Chapter 4

Mysticism and Neville Symington

The religious imperialist

Like Fromm, Neville Symington came from a conservative religious family. He became a Catholic priest but eventually abandoned God as understood in the religion of his seminary. He did not abandon religion, however. Instead, he staked out for it a vast, idiosyncratic space encompassing metaphysics, morality, psychoanalysis, interpersonal relations and a quasi-mystical understanding of 'ultimate reality'. His principal theme is that psychoanalysis *is* a religion, albeit a scientific one. It is impoverished in its current forms, Symington insists, because it has not taken possession of the core religious values taught by all the great religious reformers, the values that give life meaning. In his excellent autobiography, *A Different Path* (2016), Symington recounts that his two years of philosophical study in the seminary had a profound effect on him. Ontology became the foundation stone of his life. Ontology is a sub-discipline within metaphysics (which is a sub-discipline within philosophy) concerned with what sorts of things exist or have being. Through the study of ontology, Symington says, he came to know 'the absolute nature of existence through intellectual and emotional conviction'. Happy is the man who comes to know the absolute nature of existence. He now believed in a God who was not the God of Biblical revelation but the one elaborated by Spinoza. Later on, he 'realized that this intellectual vision had first been grasped by the seers of the Upanishads' (2016, 122). In fact, his various writings on religion support only a

DOI: 10.4324/9781003508700-4

tenuous relation to Spinoza's pantheism but do evince the influence of Eastern and Western mystics, Wilfred Bion and other British object relations theorists, particularly Donald Winnicott. To this base, he added some home-cooked metaphysics and eclectic selections from unfamiliar sources such as the Russian Orthodox Vladimir Solovyov, whom he considered the greatest of all philosophers, possibly because Solovyov preferred religious intuition over reason. Few psychoanalysts have ranged over such extensive foreign territory. Erich Fromm, whom Symington admires, had compacted religion, morality and spirituality, and proclaimed psychoanalysis a spiritual endeavor. Symington races with these ideas. Reading through his ambitious and confident prose can be a trial. He is difficult, but the philosophical expeditions are densely intertwined with his understanding of the relations between religion and psychoanalysis and cannot be ignored. Moreover, his views have become fairly representative and are often cited in the quarters of psychoanalysis under critical consideration. The philosophical and mystical conceptions he relies on are mostly untethered from mainstream learning, and his interpretations of sources are frequently eccentric. Yet Symington has real merits. He is widely read and aware that there is a vast world of learning in philosophy, theology, anthropology and history that bears on the issues that concern him. Unlike many others in the mystically inclined and spiritually sensitive schools of psychoanalysis Symington recognizes *the need to argue a case*; it is not done well, but it is exceptional that it is done at all.[1]

How does Symington arrive at the view that psychoanalysis is a scientific religion? In the opening chapters of *The Blind Man Sees* (Symington 2004), he presents several swift arguments. They are patently invalid and can be dispatched quickly. First, religion is concerned with the relations between people; psychoanalysis is concerned with relations between people; therefore psychoanalysis is a religion. One may as well argue that cats catch mice; owls catch mice; therefore, owls are cats. Second, Symington argues that Freud was a religious leader, the first 'religious leader who reversed the ancient pathway to holiness via the *fuga mundi*' (flight from the world) (2004, 20). He was a religious leader, the argument goes, because he had passed through the same tribulations as the Buddha and many saints and mystics. The premise is shaky, but even if Freud had followed a path of Awakening, Enlightenment, Struggle … Followers, and so forth, as Symington describes it, there is nothing intrinsically religious about such a path. Many thinkers and artists have passed through such trials without becoming founders of religions. And even if granted that Freud was a religious leader, it does not follow that his creation is a religion. Pythagoras *was* a religious leader, but his famous theorem and other achievements are not religious tenets.

Given Freud's posture and the predominantly atheistic ethos of later psychoanalysis, Symington knew that conflating psychoanalysis and religion might appear absurd to his readers. Nevertheless, he argues, third, that despite appearances psychoanalysis *could* be a religion because the conception of atheistic religion is sound. Thus, he says that Theravada Buddhism and Taoism, which are acknowledged as religions, are explicitly atheistic (2004, 5). The Buddha was just as much an atheist as Freud: 'theism is not an essential component of religion' (2004, 20). Recall the robust definition of religion in the previous chapter. According to it, theism is indeed not an essential feature of religions. But belief in supernatural beings such as spirits or souls, or supernatural processes such as reincarnation, preclude atheism. Moreover, even if the Buddha was a fully fledged atheist renouncing all supernatural conceptions, many, perhaps most, local expressions of Buddhism (shaped by older, underlying folk religions) are floridly supernaturalistic. Only by defining religion so broadly as to render it senseless could atheism be included under its head. Freud had warned against philosophers twisting words until they had no connection with their original meanings. The revisionary attempts at definition eventually arrive at the *laissez-faire* of 'definitional strategies' (as in Parsons 2021), where one chooses a definition that suits one's purpose best, and the concept of definition itself collapses.

There is now a burgeoning literature linking psychoanalysis to mysticism and spiritual endeavor, Freud himself to the Kabbalah and the Jewish mystical tradition, and enjoining psychotherapy as spiritual practice.[2] It is impossible in a few paragraphs, or even very many paragraphs, to cover all the territory, but a closer inspection of Symington's ideas should illuminate some of the general characteristics of this literature and demonstrate why I refer to the trend as an arc of intellectual decline. Further comments on the origins and context of this regressive trend – that of course would not be a description favored by the authors I criticize – may be found in the final chapter.

Primitive and mature religion

Symington's most consolidated essay on religion, *Emotion and Spirit* (Symington 1998), begins by distinguishing between primitive religion and mature religion. Later on, the accent falls on a distinction between primitive and natural religion. The latter distinction, seized on by several psychoanalytic writers, produces even more confusion than the first since the term 'natural religion' has for many centuries had an established meaning predicated on rational proofs of the existence of God and bears little relation to Symington's use of the term, which depends less on reason than intuition or mystical insight. Primitive religion, Symington says, is an expression of the primitive mind and its governance by the survival instinct. The instinct for survival requires the elevation and protection of the tribe – 'tribal self-magnification' – as well as obtaining protection from powerful gods through sacrifice and worship. Symington states, correctly, that the mentality underlying primitive religion still 'suffuses all the great organized religions of the world' (1998, 12).

Mature or natural religion is antithetical to primitive religion in being unbound to the survival instinct, ritual, and the formation of grandiose self-conceptions and group narcissism. How did mature religion emerge from its primitive base? Symington follows Karl Jaspers in supposing that there was an Axial Era (800 and 200 BCE) during which a number of great religious teachers radically changed mankind's religious outlook. Confucius and Lao-tzu, the Buddha, Zarathustra, the Hebrew prophets, Socrates, Plato and Aristotle make the cut; Jesus and Muhammad, who have good claims to religious innovation, are relegated in the Axial scheme (1998, 14). Symington asserts that 'All these teachers have one message in common: life's meaning is to be found in a reality beyond the immediate, beyond the senses: This reality transcends survival, and therefore the instincts which drive us towards survival' (1998, 110). That these outstanding figures had a common message is surely mistaken, but before addressing that it is worth noting how Symington, and kindred spirits before and after him, viewed religious transformation as the work of great personalities rather than, as history suggests, gradual socio-economic, moral and intellectual evolution. The idea of the great transformative religious leader, the prophet, the saint, the mystic has a singular hold on their imaginations. No gods, perhaps, but god-like figures. That the main psychoanalytic figures we are discussing here (apart from Freud) all had conservative religious upbringings may not be coincidental. It may be conjectured that Biblically repressive, possibly traumatic, childhoods had created intense needs for idealized figures to defend against persecutory internal objects.[3] In any case, for some people religious paragons become models for the conduct of life. 'What would Jesus do?' How should one live? What is it to live a morally good life? These are taxing questions indeed. Some answers lead to imitation, others to acceptance of scriptural or mystical revelation; and others to the difficult, patient work of moral reflection and philosophical investigation: several philosophical attempts at rationally grounding morality – Kantian deontology, Utilitarianism, social contract theories – have substantially shaped social and political transformations over recent centuries. Symington took the road to a syncretic mysticism.

Now, this picture of an Axial Age of religious innovators replacing primitive religion with teachings about life's meaning 'found in a reality beyond the immediate, beyond the senses' has little merit. The historical construction is an illusion. It is now recognized that Zarathustra was not a contemporary of the others but lived sometime in the 2nd millennium BCE. Much of what is characteristic of the Hebrew prophets, the exhortations to justice and righteousness, attending to the poor and powerless, dispensing with sacrifice and cult, were standard motifs almost 2,000 years earlier. Thus, a king of Lagash in the third millennium BCE proclaims himself 'the righter of social wrongs and the defender of the weak … he would never subject the waif and the widow to the powerful' (Bellah 2011, 221). Justice (Ma'at) was a principal concern of Egyptian kings. In the Egyptian Old Kingdom we hear 'I gave the hungry bread / And clothing to the naked … I rescued the weak from the strong / I gave ear to the matter of the widow' (Bellah 2011, 237). The claim that Confucius, the man Socrates or Aristotle believed that the 'meaning of life' lay in the afterlife is plainly wrong. Buddha (or his followers) founded religions, but Socrates, Plato and Aristotle, who were great moral philosophers, did not. The world of the prophets is remote from the questioning and probing of the Greek philosophers. To declare that justice should roll down like the waters and God cares not for hollow piety is a very fine thing. But it is altogether different to ask, as Socrates did tirelessly, exactly what justice and piety *are*. So, we are drawn toward distinguishing moral evolution, such as it is, a slow historical progression with multi-factor causation, from the abrupt intrusions of religious leaders. For good reason.

Religion and morality

The suggestion that the philosophers were religious innovators is tenable only on the false assumption underlying Symington's thought that religion and moral reflection are one and the same. Symington has no notion of moral reflection apart from religious reflection. In that he is consonant with the Abrahamic religions, which have conflated morality and religion. To live morally, many people believe to this day, is to live according to religious law. Since Symington's aim is to collapse morality, religion, spirituality and psychoanalysis, it is important to see at the outset that historically, and for the greater part of humanity, morality and religion have been two almost entirely different spheres.

Rules, various as they might be, relating to right conduct, loyalty, justice, obedience, respect and so forth must have antedated religions. Such conceptions are internal to any viable social group. Our Paleolithic ancestors could scarcely have survived had they not been governed by recognizably moral norms, at least as they applied within the intimate group. Hunter and gatherer societies, who may reflect our prehistory, usually have rigid moral prescriptions, but the spirits of their Animistic worlds are typically amoral, capricious, and have no moral heft (Lewis 2003, 27). In such societies, the idea that spirits should lay down laws of any kind is unknown. In ancient Mesopotamia and Egypt, conceptions of justice and right conduct were highly refined. But it was the kings, not the gods, who framed the laws and set the standards of justice and right conduct. As the Egyptologist Jan Assman said,

> justice has been in the world since time immemorial: indeed it is difficult to see how people could live together without it … In Egypt … it was situated in the human rather than divine world. Whereas the gods crave sacrificial offerings, humans crave the law. In its origins justice is something profane or secular.
>
> (Assmann 2010, 149–150)

Again, in the ancient Greek and Roman worlds, gods made neither moral nor civic law. The main function of religious practice was to keep the gods on side by performing the appropriate sacrifices and rituals. Morality, on the other hand, stood on the ground of tradition and public good sense, and laws reflecting moral norms were recognized as man-made. 'The laws', Pericles said, 'are all the rules approved and enacted by the majority in assembly, whereby they declare what ought and what ought not to be done'. They are obeyed out of deep respect, not because of fear of the gods (Bowra 1973 [1957], 81, 84).

The world changed with the accession of the Christian Roman emperors. But we can now see that there are only contingent conceptual and historical connections between morality and religion. Having conflated the two, Symington is obliged to provide some content for morality to illuminate what he thinks religion is. Morality and religion, one and the same, aim at the good. What is the good that morality, religion *and* psychoanalysis should aim at? To fill in the required content, Symington consults a number of philosophers, mystics and the Upanishads, but initially Socrates – a good man to go to – devoting an entire chapter to him. Unfortunately, Symington's Socrates is a creature entirely of his own fancy, bearing almost no relation to what we know about the man. The fancies, however, point directly to his own views. According to Symington, Socrates challenged the primitive religion current in Greece, and what he taught 'implied that the worship of the gods who sanctioned the political ideologies of Athenian life should be renounced' (Symington 1996, 41). Socrates was 'concerned to teach what is right and wrong', but because his principles were not organized by a faith community it is 'more accurate to call the doctrine of Socrates a spirituality than a religion' (1996, 38). 'The good', according to Socrates, is something definite but not concrete; it is real but 'can only be grasped through psychic action'; as a 'spiritual quality', the good 'must be grasped through a realization of the inner eye' (1996, 40). In rejecting the identity of the good with pleasure, Socrates believed that the 'good is known through conscience and in an act of judgement' (1996, 42). Socrates was greater than Buddha or Jesus because he established a spirituality based on reason. 'On the criterion we have adopted for distinguishing between primitive and mature religion, this makes Socrates one of the great spiritual leaders of mankind' (1996, 41).

None of this is true of Socrates, and what appear to be psychological twists on later Platonic doctrines distort them beyond recognition. Socrates was a religious conservative, very exacting, Xenophon tells us, about observing traditional rites and sacrifices. He could scarcely be accused of teaching 'the good' for man, persistently professing not to know it. However, Symington obscurely senses an important Socratic achievement: he was probably the first to apply philosophical methods to ethics, and he shifted the focus of Greek philosophy from the natural world to the nature of man. He argued something like this: The goodness of anything is its fitness to perform its proper function. The goodness of a knife, for example, is its ability to cut well, cutting being the function of a knife. So, what is goodness for man? What is the specific excellence of man? To determine that requires that we know ourselves, for with knowledge of ourselves will come knowledge of the good for man. In seeking to know the nature of man – of humanity – it is unlikely that Socrates was enjoining introspection, possibly in the manner of the Delphic maxim 'Know thyself', though he certainly thought that knowing one's own ignorance was a good start. To Symington's primed ear, however, Socratic injunctions about seeking self-knowledge sound both spiritual and psychoanalytic.

The road to spirituality

Satisfied that morality and religion are one, and believing that he has Socrates on side with the idea of 'the good' for man as a 'spiritual quality' grasped by 'psychic action' and 'the inner eye', Symington's next objective is to link the religious to the spiritual and to psychoanalysis. The argument goes like this. The moral perspective is a religious perspective. Religion exists in the emotional space between persons, and 'the recognition the "other" has a claim on me is the religious attitude of mind … The work of creating the full reality of a personal relationship is the religious task' (1998, 43). The highest gear of religion is the spiritual, and since religion incorporates morality 'true spirituality incorporates the moral' (1998, 46). But what is spirituality? 'Spirituality is that mental discipline whose goal is the purification of moral action' (1998, 47). 'A spiritual person is one who makes the good an internal possession … The person who is in search of the motive that drives his actions in order to purify his intentions is engaged in spiritual activity' (1998, 172). This congenial connection between spirituality and interest in understanding one's motives, purifying them, avoiding self-deception, insincerity and so forth, is surely artificial and counterfactual. Many of the wicked and unregenerate atheists have these interests also. Freud may be spiritual in Symington's estimation, but Nietzsche or Sartre? But to proceed to the conclusion: psychoanalysis is deeply concerned with actions and intentions, with, so to speak, 'purifying' them, and:

> if we follow [Karl] Abraham in saying that the goal of psychoanalysis is the strengthening of character, then we must define such an analysis as having as its aim the transformation of bad actions into good; an analysis is successful to the extent that it is able to do this … If the goal of psychoanalysis is the transformation of bad actions into good, is it not right to call this a spiritual aim?
>
> (Symington 1998, 181).

Well, if the aim of psychoanalysis is to transform bad actions into good then, presumably, the analyst knows what 'the good' is and how to recognize it. Superficially, this may appear unproblematic; it may appear unproblematic to psychotherapists practicing suggestion or on the cusp of transformation into gurus. What ordinary people would call virtues, such as humility, courage, candor are good; the vices, such as egotism, greed and injustice, are bad. But Symington knows that this is problematic. How do we *know* what is good apart from culture-relative consensus? How do we justify our judgments? At this problematic point, Symington's conception of *conscience* assumes inordinate importance. His conception of conscience is not to be confused with aspects of the Freudian ego-ideal or superego. It seems to be conceived as something innate and responsible for an innate ability to distinguish good and evil: 'we all have within us a categorization of good and evil' (1998, 111). Here I must reproduce two lengthy passages because an exposition of Symington's thought without them would be difficult and improbable.

> When I listen to my conscience I am attentive to a principle within me but at the same time extends beyond me. It is *in* me but it is not *just* me; something has a claim on me which is at the same time greater than me. It is difficult to avoid the conclusion that conscience speaks for that reality whose praises were sung by the seers of the Upanishads. The seers comprehended this reality and meditated upon it … The Buddha stressed meditation … but his realization that conscience was the organ of reality gave his truth a practical application which had been lacking in a refined way within Hinduism … Socrates did not unify the pursuit of the good with the comprehension of reality. To act according to conscience is to pursue the good. The apprehension of the truth is through an act of intellect. The pursuit of the good is through moral action. When the truth and the good are understood to coincide we have religion.
>
> (1998, 155–156).

> The virtuous act is an action of the ego which frees split parts from captivity, from being agents of the vicious personalities, and brings them into unity … At the same time conscience makes itself heard. It is the voice beckoning the virtuous act.

> The virtuous act integrates the ego parts. A product of integration of the ego-parts is self-knowledge; therefore the virtuous act is the prerequisite for self-knowledge … If it is accurate to say that the goal of psychoanalysis is self-knowledge, and if our argument is right that self-knowledge is dependent upon the virtuous act, then the process of psychoanalysis is a spirituality … We are forced to conclude that psychoanalysis is a religion as well as a spirituality.
>
> (1998, 167–169)

I believe that the key ideas in these passages are unsalvageable, but we are obliged to try to make some sense of them. Similar ideas are espoused by thinkers who have taken ancient and medieval texts all too seriously, mixed them with psychoanalytic conceptions, and mistaken obscurity for light.[4] There appear to be three main strands of thought competing in these passages.

The first is psychoanalytic in complexion. Symington takes it that the ego is not unitary but composed of fragments, which can be in mutual antagonism. He is surely right that 'it is an inherent belief of psychoanalysis that to own different parts of ourselves is a good thing in itself' (1998, 174). Actions that disintegrate the self are generally bad, at least for that self. He goes on to explain that 'fragments in relation are the source of good actions, those in antagonism are the source of bad actions' (1998, 180). It is hard to see why that should be so. Perhaps Symington's thought is that acting with self-knowledge that is the product of an integrated self is more likely to lead to good actions than bad. That may be true, but it would seem to make the morality of an action entirely dependent on its source and ignore its consequences, a hardly satisfactory conclusion. Many philosophers believe reasonably that the consequences of an action are as, or more, important morally than its motives. One of Symington's key propositions is that 'the virtuous act integrates ego parts'. It is from this proposition that he concludes that psychoanalysis is a religion and a spirituality, but it doesn't follow from any other premises he presents. The argument is: virtuous acts lead to self-integration, self-integration to self-knowledge, and self-knowledge being the aim of psychoanalysis is what renders it spiritual. But it is difficult at the first step to see why a person's acting virtuously – dutifully, generously, courageously, or maximizing happiness for all – should lead to an integration of their ego. Without the first, unsupported premise the argument collapses. So we have yet another failed argument for the equation of religion, spirituality and psychoanalysis.

The second strand of Symington's reasoning concerns conscience. The novel and peculiar idea that conscience is an 'organ of reality' beckoning toward the good goes beyond, I think, most Christian conceptions of God-implanted conscience and, of course, well beyond Freud's conception of the mature superego, which, Freud lamented, was rather scarcely distributed. It is convenient to be able to invoke an organ speaking for reality and beckoning toward virtuous acts that integrate the ego. Only, one wonders, if all of humanity has this useful organ, why are so many immoral backsliders, and why is the organ so culturally promiscuous? If conscience is in possession of the good, as it must be if it beckons toward it, Symington should plainly tell us in respectable detail what the good for man is. This much seems clear: the introduction of conscience in Symington's sense looks like an artificial device to advance an argument. But even if there were such a thing providing moral guidance, integrating the self in its light cannot be all there is to human virtue.

The third thread is derived from the Upanishads, though probably fortified by the metaphysical views of Wilfred Bion, to whom we soon turn. At this point, religion and psychoanalysis are subordinated to an ancient mystical metaphysics. The reality 'sung by the seers', as Symington phrases it, is ultimate reality. When he speaks of a person, the other, Symington says, he is referring to

> the *being* of the other, and ontological reflection tells me that *being* is one and indivisible. It is therefore the reality in which I and the other share, and is the root upon which the concept of transference is based … This being is identical with that reality apprehended by the seers whose metaphysical insights have been recorded in the *Upanishads*.
>
> (Symington 2004, 76)

The thought seems to be that because all humanity is part of the unity of ultimate reality, that fact creates *moral* bonds between persons and between persons and nature. 'The reality in which I and the entire human community participate has an ultimate value, and this has a claim upon me. My manner of acting towards myself and others is therefore the central concern of mature religion' (1998, 147). This sharing or identification with others, and with ultimate reality, or at least the recognition of this mutuality, Symington calls 'participated being'. In medieval fashion he argues that everything there is has a common predicate 'existent'.[5] We all exist and are therefore part of an ultimate reality that is indivisible. THAT THOU ART, says Symington, says it all (2004, 78). Perhaps a formula common in Gnostic and Neoplatonic literature of late antiquity says it better, as in the remarkable passage: 'I am Thou and Thou art I: where Thou art, there am I also. I am disposed in all things: wherever Thou wilt, Thou dost assemble me, and in assembling me thou dost assemble thyself' (Dodds 1965, 73).

Well, this is high metaphysics indeed. Ontological reflection has told Symington that *being* (the universe?) is one and indivisible. Let's put this bold claim to one side for the moment. The question then is why participating with others in ultimate reality should create moral bonds. After all, being born into the world does not confer set sympathies and is not like joining a club or moral community with mutually agreed obligations. A vision of common humanity, of recognizing oneself in the other, our shared fate, is a noble vision. It is unfortunately all too obvious that establishing moral bonds requires more than such a vision. It is wishful thinking to imagine that this metaphysical principle could sustain a universal or even a local moral order. Yet from this slender metaphysical base Symington proceeds to draw out many moral and practical implications for psychoanalysis. Acting according to the principle that participated being has a claim upon me is the ground of mature religion and therefore of psychoanalysis (2004, 77ff). Conscience is 'a signal from participated being'. The obtaining of participated being is the guarantor of mental health. The obliteration of participated being is the source of psychopathology. Uncovering the processes that lead to this obliteration is *the* psychoanalytic process. Psychopathology has its roots in narcissism, the love of oneself to the exclusion of others, which is alienation from participated being. The core of the human condition is narcissism, and the aim of psychoanalysis is rescuing the individual from the human condition by means of 'soul analysis' (1998, 117). There is much more in this vein that must be omitted. What has gone wrong is reasonably clear. Symington's religious and moral preoccupations have led him into an untenable metaphysics that has in turn distorted his understanding of psychoanalysis. The metaphysical prism is distorting the clinical realities. *Psychoanalytic psychology is placed on a metaphysical foundation much less secure than the psychology itself.* That is a regressive result. And now we must ask more precisely how we got here.

Mysticism

First, the Upanishadic context. Perhaps this much can be safely said (by a non-expert like the present author) that Hindu philosophy, even its earliest expressions, is a mixture of rationalistic and mystical elements, and Symington was influenced more by the latter than the former. Three principles in this area of his work stand out. Symington accepts, as an unquestioned fact, a deep-going distinction between appearance and reality. At the common-sense level, the distinction is natural enough. The moon appears to be small, but in reality it is large. The stick in the water appears bent, but in reality is straight. In the dream state, dreams appear real, but are not. An apple has phenomenal properties, but behind those we perceive there must be some substratum in which the properties inhere. Arguing along these lines, some philosophers in both Eastern and Western traditions have suggested that we may (almost) be inescapably mired in a much deeper appearance–reality distinction: perhaps we *never* can perceive anything but appearances. The most influential expression of this view is the myth of Plato's cave, in which bound prisoners can perceive on the walls only the shadows of real objects paraded behind them. Some readers will recognize various ideas that have been introduced into psychoanalysis as descendants of these conceptions: Bion's O, the unknown or incommunicable self, 'the unknowable ground of creativity as such', and so forth. Symington uses Kantian language in the passage below, but the inspiration is the Upanishads, in the distinction between the veil of *maya* or illusion drawn over *brahman*, ultimate reality.

> Whereas we know this [phenomenal] manifestation of reality through the senses we only know reality itself through an act of intuition. It is the diverse character of reality that is known through the senses, but its unity which is its essential nature is only known through insight. [The] Upanishadic seers were the first human beings to pierce through the *phenomenon* to the *noumenon* … these seers intuited Ultimate Reality from its sensuous encasement.
>
> (Symington 1998, 29)

It is interesting that in the West, the deep-going appearance–reality distinction precipitated a variety of reactions from the Greek Sophists onwards, and acutely after Descartes set the epistemological agenda for modern philosophy. These included various forms of skepticism, phenomenalism, idealism and Kant's transcendental idealism; as well as Realist rejections of the distinction, predominant today. But the idea that rather mysterious acts of intuition or insight could penetrate through the veil of appearance to ultimate reality, or to God, seems to have remained a marginal affair, the property of Gnostics and mystics. Hindu thought, or at least some schools of it, have been more accommodating to the idea that one can peep behind the veil by means of some special intuition or mystical experience of the sort that Symington seems to claim for himself. The second principle, then, is that ultimate reality, the thing behind the veil of appearance or illusion, can be directly intuited or experienced. This is a strange conception. What could it be to experience ultimate reality? One might have thought that ultimate reality has something to do with quarks and quantum loops, space-time and so forth, explored using complex mathematics, observation and experimentation. Are we to suppose that the ancient sages and mystics were able to penetrate to ultimate reality with the few resources available to them? It is clear that they experienced *something*, but that something is mischaracterized as ultimate reality. Perhaps they mistook serenity for reality?

The third principle, implicit in Symington's view of participated being, is that ultimate reality is infinite, an interconnected whole, a unity – an Absolute, as this cluster of notions tends to be described. This insight about the nature of the universe is supposed to be one of the fruits of the mystical intuition or experience. It is a report of the mystic's accomplishment. It may be that this ambitious and totalistic language – infinity, unity, ultimate reality, Absolute – is not strictly necessary to ground the main conceptions of 'spiritually sensitive psychoanalysis' of which Symington is a forerunner, and perhaps of those psychoanalytic thinkers who lean on Eastern traditions, but it is favored by them. Thus, Lev, in his manifesto of the spiritually sensitive psychoanalysis movement, tells us that the Absolute is beyond the myriad phenomena that humans face in the material world, that all things in the universe are interconnected and that the universe is 'a unity that is intelligent, self-organized and ever-evolving … imbued with a consciousness or life-force' (Lev 2023, 5). There is an old joke about the Holy Roman Empire being neither holy, Roman nor an Empire. Some of our best contemporary physics and philosophy is telling us that at the most basic level the universe is granular (rather as Democritus thought) and that it can't be infinite or 'self-evolving' (if it sprang from the 'Big Bang') and is possibly only one of many universes. But the greater difficulty is to *make sense* of these notions of the Absolute. Does the universe being interconnected and imbued with consciousness mean that when I sneeze the weather on Venus changes and that bricks are conscious? Extraordinary claims about a holistic universe cannot be assumed; they need to be established coherently, possibly by drawing on the heavy armaments of Idealistic thought. So far, it seems, the mystically and spiritually inclined schools have deployed only butter knives.[6]

Symington, at any rate, believed that acts of intuition or mystical insight can reveal an ultimate reality behind transient appearances that is infinite, whole and Absolute. How does mystical insight, religious experience or intuition acquire this information about ultimate reality? Gershom Scholem (1995 [1946]) repeatedly emphasized that there are no mystical traditions outside religious ones. It might be more correct to say, alluding to Eastern traditions, that there are no mystical traditions outside some religious or philosophical framework. Thus, in *The Analyst and the Mystic*, Sudhir Kakar explains that

> Upanishadic mysticism ... is a quest for spiritual illumination wherein a person's deepest essence is discovered to be identical with the common source of all other animate and inanimate beings. Yogic mysticism strives to realize the immortality of the soul outside time, space and matter ... In both Upanishadic and Yogic mysticism there is no trace of love or of yearning for communion with God ... It is only in *bhakti* or devotional mysticism... where love for the Deity creeps in, where the mystic's soul or 'self' is finally united with God (or Goddess) in an ecstatic surrender, that Hindu mysticism exhibits a strong family resemblance to the mysticism of monotheistic faiths.
>
> (Kakar 2007, 3)

In *The Inner World* (2012), Kakar explains that in Hindu culture the ultimate aim of existence is *Moksha*, roughly translated as transcendence, self-realization or salvation, 'when all distinctions between subject and object have been transcended, a direct experience of the fundamental unity of human being with the infinite' (2012, 19). This is not 'a temporary surge of oceanic feeling, but a constant and fully aware living-in-the-ocean' (2012, 20). 'Reality, according to Hindu belief, can be apprehended or known only through those archaic, unconscious, pre-verbal processes of sensing and feeling ... which are thought to be in touch with the fundamental rhythms and harmonies of the universe' (2012, 23).

It is a good conjecture that what Symington experienced, or was gesturing toward, felt something like *Moksha*, salvation through 'a direct experience of the fundamental unity of human being with the infinite'. Now, Kakar provides what Symington had not, the rudiments of an answer to our question: How is it possible for mystical experience or intuition to provide information about ultimate reality? That answer will be shown to fail. Then we can briefly consider another objection that would appear to undermine all mystical projects.

Notice that achieving insight about ultimate reality, or the immortality of the soul, is not the end result of a process of reasoning. According to Kakar, ultimate reality can be apprehended mystically because archaic, unconscious, pre-verbal processes are 'in touch with the fundamental rhythms and harmonies of the universe'. How does that work? Human beings are clusters of organic cells. Can it be that these fragile, ephemeral things are in touch with the fundamental rhythms, the mighty beat of the universe? What *are* the fundamental rhythms of the universe? Such communication between man and universe would presuppose some sort of preestablished harmony unknown to physics or physiology. It *presupposes* the picture of participated being, of the interconnected Absolute, and related conceptions. But this picture of an interconnected ultimate reality is supposed to be *revealed*, and evidentially supported by, mystical experience. Mystical experience understood as acquiring knowledge, as having cognitive content of some sort, presupposes the very metaphysical or religious conceptions which are supposed to be justified by the mystical experience. That is fatal to the epistemology of most mystical endeavors. The argument does not touch contentless mystical experience, the apophatic ways, or the views of those who are comfortable with meaningless phrases, logical contradictions and ineffable ways of knowing.[7]

A second argument penetrates further. It is perhaps conceivable that there are mental states lacking conscious cognitive and affective content, lacking even a background of unconscious phantasy (Damasio 2010). Some such states may emerge at certain points in a meditative cycle, or mindfulness, or experiencing union with gods, and may have therapeutic value. But if the mystical experience has content and points beyond itself, then it is invariably embedded in the supernatural context of one religious or philosophical tradition or another. And here's the rub. The different traditions report different and incompatible supernatural realities. The shaman's soul leaves his body and travels to a nether world, returning with reports of animal spirits and enemy shamans. Ezekiel has a vision of God on a chariot throne of lapis lazuli; the Apostle John sees God on a throne of jasper encircled by an emerald rainbow. Julian of Norwich has equivocal encounters with Jesus. Ramakrishna embraces the goddess Kali, and the Upanishadic sages and Neville Symington experience ultimate reality. It is difficult to reconcile these reports and, of course, many others of the kind. They cannot all be true because some are flatly incompatible. The Jewish mystic must say that the Hindu mystic gets it wrong: Ramakrishna could not have embraced Kali because there is no Kali. And of course, the reverse holds. The best conclusion to draw is that none of the reports are true, on pain of indefensible religious chauvinism.[8]

These matters require more detailed discussion than can be included here, but perhaps enough has been said to cast serious doubt on the evidential credentials of mystical or spiritual experience. As sources of knowledge about their objects, they have little if any warrant. But such experiences can, of course, reveal a great deal about the person who has them, about the culture in which that person is situated, and the people who take the experiences to be epistemically significant. And at the meditational and saintly end of the spectrum it seems likely that they do have beneficial, therapeutic effects, at least in the medical understanding of these terms.

Finally, there is a discussion about whether mystical or spiritual experiences are regressive or *sui generis*, irreducible, and if *sui generis*, then possibly transcendent. Freud's reductive approach to the so-called oceanic feeling has come under blanket fire from major figures such as Erik Erikson. But the crux does not appear to have been well articulated. Proponents of irreducibility would be safer to insist, not that all mystical experience is irreducible to regressive states, but that it is *possible* that some may be. Whether a particular mental state is regressive or not is an empirical issue to be determined case by case. The traditional psychoanalytic presumption in favor of regression arises from its skepticism about mysticism and divinity. The experiential content of the mystical state comes from somewhere, and if it is not in fact the experience of something transcendent, then it is not unreasonable to conclude that the content is regressive material. There is much evidence that points in this direction. But even if it were demonstrable that at least *some* mystical states do not evince regressive material, it is drawing a very long bow indeed to infer a new psychodynamic position, a transcendent or contemplative position (Black 2006a; Lev 2023), that goes beyond the fact that we are creatures with imagination as well as thinking reeds.

A critical note on Wilfred Bion

Bion's theoretical work is problematic philosophically and to the best of my knowledge has not, unlike Freud's or Klein's or Lacan's, been taken up by either professional philosophers or scientists. (I stand to be corrected.) Apart from the therapeutic community it has attracted the attention of religious thinkers and people interested in mysticism and the occult. The reason for the philosophical and scientific neglect appears to be twofold. The metaphysics which it proposes to underwrite psychoanalytic processes is bad metaphysics; and, worse, Bion makes no serious attempt to propound or defend it. He presents a series of asseverations instead, as if they stated the incontestable. The net effect is to weaken the psychoanalytic psychology of his concern, which is, in fact, in much better shape than the metaphysics on which he hoped to base it. One suspects that Bion's influence has more to do with his justly admired clinical acumen than his metaphysics or overarching subjective metapsychology, a 'psychical mathematics' that was doomed at the outset.[9] He contributed very little directly to the understanding of religion but, like Winnicott, created an array of conceptions that have encouraged others who are motivated to reconcile religion and mystical notions with psychoanalysis, or, rather, to subordinate the latter to the former.

Bion is an allusive and elusive writer. At the center of his metaphysics is the concept of 'O' which designates 'ultimate reality, absolute truth, the godhead, the infinite, the thing-in-itself'. Some followers have amplified the conception by adding inherent pre-conceptions, Ideal (Platonic) forms, chaos, *Ananke* and other curious items (Grotstein 2009, 335; Eigen 1998, 39–40). This is quite the ontological slum. I will only consider briefly the widespread assumption that O is the same as Kant's notion of noumena, a notion that seems to enjoy respect in the psychoanalytic community. Bion explicitly aligns himself with Kant, stating that O, like 'things-in themselves', refer to objects that are unknowable to mankind (Bion 2023 [1962], 10). But that alignment can't possibly be right. Bion states that O can be felt and evolve and become an object of K (knowledge). That is impossible in the Kantian scheme of transcendental idealism. Noumena cannot be felt or evolve (Strawson 1966).

But then Bion says that the examples of O he provides are only intended to allude to *his* meaning (Bion 1970, 87). So, perhaps, the identity with noumena is not intended to be complete. In any event, Bion accepts the deep-going appearance–reality distinction of which the Kantian case is an instance, and states that

> in any object, material or immaterial, resides the unknowable ultimate reality, the 'thing-in-itself'. Objects have *emanations or emergent qualities* or evolving characteristics that impinge upon the human personality as phenomena. Of these qualities the personality may be consciously aware; they differ from the ultimate reality.
>
> (Bion 1970, 87. My italics)

This is partly Kantian, of course, but compounded with a Neoplatonic theory of emanations, discernible in some Kabbalistic works, that Kant would have found amusing. Bion clearly responded to these prescientific and mystical notions very seriously and detrimentally. According to Michael Eigen, Bion said to him, 'I use the Kabbalah as a framework for psychoanalysis' (Govrin 2016, 136). One may as well build a rocket to Mars using Aristotelian physics.

I think I have said enough about the metaphysics of mysticism above, and I want now to complete this brief opinionated note by drawing attention to Bion's warrantless epistemology. Bion says that

> [O] stands for absolute truth in and of any object: it is assumed that this cannot be known about a human being; it can be known about, its presence can be recognized and felt, but it cannot be known. It is possible to be at one with it. That it exists is an essential postulate of science but it cannot be scientifically discovered. No psychoanalytic discovery is possible without recognition of its existence, at-one-ment with it and evolution. The religious mystics have probably approximated most closely to the experience of it. Its existence is as essential to science as to religion.
>
> (Bion 1970, 30)

Suppose we overlook the contradictions and category mistakes in this passage and question how Bion arrived at the view that O is an essential postulate of science that cannot be scientifically discovered. What are his grounds for maintaining that O's existence is essential to science, as essential as to religion? The claims are not self-evident; in fact, nothing like the notion of O appears in contemporary physics, anthropology, neuroscience, geology or entomology. Bion does not provide (so far as I know) any reasoned argument for believing that O is an essential postulate of any science. It is difficult to see how psychoanalytic experience provides grounds for his claim. That will be disputed. But, in any case, psychoanalysts and therapists *do* make discoveries without recourse to Bion's 'essential postulate', and appear to be able to work without it. Bion's mystical metaphysics is a strange, unsupported structure. It was constructed before the great explosion of neuroscientific and materialistic conceptions of mind that occurred in the last quarter of the 20th century. It would seem that, being at the mercy of the few philosophical ideas he encountered, he cobbled together the metaphysics and thought it was the only game in town; he believed that mystics were holding good hands.

Notes

1 The therapists referred to as belonging to 'mystical' or 'spiritually sensitive' schools, to which (in some instances) could be added those who employ meditative techniques derived from Buddhist or Hindu practices, form a heterogeneous grouping. The evident commonalities are religious backgrounds informing them, and belief in supernaturalistic conceptions of reality and epistemic access to such reality through direct or immediate forms of experience.

2 Apart from the works discussed below, the following may be included: Pickering 2019; Pearson and Marlo (eds) 2020; Bar Ness 2021.

3 Donald Capps argues that religion is 'inherently disposed toward the abuse of children' because it provides theological legitimation for the punishment of children and promotes ideas and beliefs that are 'inherently tormenting to them' (Capps 1995, xi). The idea that children come into the world sinful and require to have their wills broken is part and parcel of Biblical literalism. Punitive attitudes often found in the religious household are seen as Biblically endorsed. It has been noted that Protestant Christians who advocate harsh physical punishment tend to be intensely apocalyptic. For the child impending beatings

loom as catastrophe, the end of the world. Paranoia may also be conditioned by child abuse, laying the groundwork for anticipation of attack and harm. People whose wills have been broken often become paranoid. Capps maintains that 'religious ideas may be as abusive as the physical punishment of children' (xi). Doctrines of hell and eternal punishment, aversive attitudes towards natural sexual feeling, the breaches between friends occasioned by religious segregation can cause great emotional torment to a child. Richard Dawkins (2006, 318) cites the case of Pastor Robert's hell-houses, which contain frightening representations of infernal punishments designed to deter 12-year-olds from sin. Capps proposes that physical and emotional abuse operates traumatically in much the same way as child sexual abuse. Consequent to trauma there is repression of the traumatic experience which leads to dissociation of part of the self which is intricated in the experience, a withdrawal of feeling or affect and the frequently observed loss of confidence in their own judgement that victims suffer. Hence, Capps observes, people who can think independently and well about politics, science, etc. become unexpectedly bland, uncritical and deferential about religion (Capps 1995, 52–53).

4 For example, Bion 1970; Eigen 1998; Rubin 2006; Cunningham 2006; Lev 2023 who provides a long list of sympathetic works in his opening chapter. The mystical texts are, of course, of great historical interest and their mesmerizing allure is of great psychoanalytic interest.

5 The idea that existence is a predicate was refuted by Kant; it's not being a predicate underlies modern logic of first order predicate calculus.

6 Around the turn of the 19th century British philosophy was dominated by F. H. Bradley's Absolute Idealism and to a lesser extent by a number of related Hegelian doctrines. Bradley's was an imposing and respectable edifice. Crucial to it was his 'doctrine of internal relations' which vouchsafed, so to speak, the Absoluteness and interconnectedness of it all. The doctrine was dismantled by Bertrand Russell and G. E. Moore, giving birth in the process to Analytic philosophy, a mirror opposite of Absolute Idealism, that still dominates Anglophone and Scandinavian philosophy. I believe there are very few philosophers today in the halls of academia who entertain the notion that the universe is some sort of unity imbued with consciousness or spirit.

7 See, e.g., Jones 2002; Pickering 2019.

8 Arguments undermining the epistemological value of religious experience are detailed in Mackie 1982; Gale 1993.

9 For the inevitable failure of 'subjective metapsychology' see Davidson's classic 'Mental events' and 'Psychology as philosophy' in Davidson 1980. Bion states that in psychoanalysis 'all theory must find its origin within the subjective experiences of the clinical encounter'. One wonders why that must be so? Freud drew on biology, anthropology, infant observation and the incipient neurosciences of his day, and, of course, infant observation and neurobiology today are rich sources of theory.

Chapter 5

Psychoanalysis and spirituality, sacred and profane

A narrative of resurgence

There is a narrative about the relations between psychoanalysis, religion and spirituality that goes something like this. Freud was an uncompromising atheist, as were most of his immediate circle and several generations that followed them. For most of the 20th century, psychoanalysts were hostile or indifferent to religion and insensitive to the religious or spiritual concerns of their patients. The two main reasons for that, the narrative goes, were the shadow cast by Freud and, at least in the United States, the determination of psychoanalysts to see their discipline as strictly medical and scientific. The evidence presented for these claims is the paucity of psychoanalytic publications about the religious and spiritual aspects of the self until late into the century. Of course, there were major outliers such as Jung, Erich Fromm and Erik Erikson, but it is probably true that, by and large, psychoanalysts were not especially concerned with these transcendental matters. Whether that was because of psychoanalytic animus toward such matters or because the devoutly religious were taking their emotional turmoil to confessors, pastors and the many institutions that religions provide for accommodating distress seems to me a moot issue. In any event, the narrative continues, a number of influential analysts – Donald Winnicott, Hans Loewald, Stephen Mitchell and others – had started the process of readjusting psychoanalytic focus from negative symptoms to nurturing of the patient's capacity for creativity, authenticity and openness to

DOI: 10.4324/9781003508700-5

experience; normative matters to be sure, which sound as if they entail moral or spiritual attainments. Then, quite suddenly, in the first decades of the 21st century, in 'a Copernican revolution' or 'paradigm shift', a tide of psychoanalytic publications emerged sensitive to religious and spiritual concerns. And so, today, analysts 'do not hesitate to delve into each and every aspect and branch of religious, spiritual and mystical occupation … They even write about parapsychology and about magic' (Lev 2023, 2). We have heralds of a 'spiritually sensitive psychoanalysis'.

Moreover, as if by coincidence, the world in the last few decades experienced a massive revival of religion and spirituality, traditional and profane. Spiritually sensitive psychoanalysis, accommodating and respectful of these concerns, stands ready for this market.

That is the narrative we must now probe. It needs to be recalled that historically the resting state of humankind has been religion in one form or another. Nevertheless, there does appear to be a revival of religious profession and spiritual hankering in recent decades. It is uneven and it is hard to know what to make of it. In educated Western Europe, Canada and Australia atheism is on the rise, but in the United States heartland and in Eastern Europe and Russia aggressive Christianity is on the rise. In Islamic nations fundamentalism is on the rise. But the profession of religion is no guarantee of it. In Australia, for example, the numbers professing religious commitment are relatively high, but only about 9% are church-goers. And the faithful are discriminating. Denial of Divinity or the Resurrection is no longer considered an obstacle to Christian affiliation. In the United Kingdom 15% of people identifying as Christians don't believe in God. Still, in the United States, Africa, South America, Russia and many Islamic nations a revival of religion seems unequivocal.

The revival may be considered in three overlapping parts. 'New Age Spirituality' is almost antique now, but in the West still has an enthusiastic following. Per Granqvist defines the movement as possessing 'a wide range of beliefs and activities that typically combine occultism, astrology, parapsychology, alternative (holistic, complementary) medicine, certain outgrowths of humanist psychology, and modifications of Eastern thinking imported into a Western context' (Granqvist 2020, 212). 'In contrast to religion', he says, 'the New Age movement does not typically provide an attachment figure at its doctrinal "center". Any center to speak of is the unreserved "celebration of the self"' (2020, 214). The absence of attachment figures seems paradoxical in the light of our understanding, but only until a given context. These various expressions of irrationalism tend to create circles. The Kabbalah, Hermetic texts, Rosicrucianism, astrology, alternative medicine, and similar expressions attract study, ritual and self-healing groups who become attachment objects. Spiritual and fringe therapies with their colorful accessories (crystals, candles, homeopathic tinctures) have a booming market and often orbit around particular stores or individuals. And some of the fascination with the occult is crystallized in following movies and internet influencers. Harry Potter is an institution. Christian and Eastern sects and cults offering belonging and rehabilitation, often only perversely related to the original founders, are prospering. Scientology has entered the mainstream. Some of the folk who visit Druidic and pagan sites presumably have spiritual beliefs, although how much of it is just fun is hard to say. This development is one aspect of the spiritual revival.

The second aspect is the growth of Pentecostalism, understood as including various charismatic groups. There are over 600 million members worldwide, and projected to be a billion by 2050. It is easily the fastest growing of all religions. To what does Pentecostalism owe its allure? Alaistair McGrath, the prolific scourge of atheism who was among the first to notice this phenomenon, describes it this way:

> Although Pentecostalism can be thought of as traditionalist in its Christian theology, it differs radically from other Christian groupings in placing emphasis on speaking in tongues and its highly experiential forms of worship, which involve prophesying, healings and exorcisms. A direct, transforming, personal encounter with God is seen as a normal feature of the Christian life … Pentecostalism stresses a direct, immediate experience of God and avoids the rather dry and cerebral forms of Christianity which many find unattractive and unintelligible.
>
> (McGrath 2004, 194–195)

McGrath thinks that because it is 'experiential' and based on the immediacy of 'God's presence through the Holy Spirit' rather than on the study of texts Pentecostalism escapes many of the criticisms and pesky philosophical objections leveled at traditional Christian theologies. Its style of worship and lack of intellectual sophistication have made Pentecostalism very effective in communicating its message and bridging cultural gaps. It is a great force in Africa where, according to McGrath, people are intimately in touch with spiritual reality.

> Many villagers throughout the region are highly aware of spiritual forces, which they often seek to consult and control through a complex system of divinations, charms and spells. With the arrival of Christianity, these spiritual forces are understood to have been tamed or conquered – though not eliminated – through the death and resurrection of Christ. The Christian gospel is interpreted in terms of deliverance from spiritual oppression, release from the power of curses, and liberation from the baleful influence of ancestors.
>
> (McGrath 2004, 205–206)[1]

That is the second aspect of the 'spiritual' revival in the West: retreat from rationality, resurgence of superstition, spirit possession and omnipotent or 'magical' modes of experience and thought. There are, of course, other developments specific to nations and circumstances and the most baleful of these is the third aspect of the revival. Fascism has been described by Hannah Arendt as the affiliation of capital, state and church. The recent developments in the United States evidently have complex causes, but the result is unquestionable: an incipient, destructive, religiously driven fascism unrestrained by scruple of law or truth.[2] President Trump is undoubtedly a malignant narcissist who has injected into American society louring violence, debased discourse and hatred of truth that may fragment it irreparably and contaminate the globe (Kernberg 2023). That his undisguised deceitfulness, grandiosity and shamelessness gives shape and purpose to his mainly Christian constituency appears paradoxical, but only on the face of it. The ground was fertile. The white Christian nationalism he opportunistically champions is unconnected to love of country. In the annals of American exceptionalism, white American Christians were once the chosen people, the light on the hill, but have since been dispossessed (starting with the civil rights legislation of the 1960s, in Trumpian discourse) and must now resume their rightful place of superiority. Trump and his enablers exploit the religious disposition of the nation and the narcissistic wounds that have been festering for decades.[3] Day by day, the American polity is taking on the conformations of religious totalitarianism.

I suspect that these developments are not what the enthusiasts of religious and spiritual revival in psychoanalysis have in mind. Theirs, I think, is a more tender vision. They speak of therapeutic sensitivity, embrace of religious and spiritual values, and of furthering their patients' spiritual growth and moral ideals; indeed, rather as if they were moralists or gurus, not psychoanalysts. Perhaps also they have in mind the mild and pacific embodiments of Buddhism and the various meditational and spiritual techniques enjoined by some psychotherapists, or the joys of religious community and the ecstasies and serenities of the mystics. Yet it seems to me that the harsh reality of the religious and spiritual revival I described eclipses these fragile and equivocal things. Moral and intellectual clarity and compassion are not the salient features of *that* revival.

Let me return to some remarks made in Chapter 1. We noticed there that mystical attempts at building psychological bridges between man and deity appear to peak in times of social distress. This was so in Egypt and Mesopotamia during the collapse of the Bronze Age empires, in Greece in the aftermath of the Peloponnesian War. Christianity consolidated in the misery of the 3rd century CE when the new urban centers of migration failed to provide the previous security of family, clan and locality. The most imaginative works of Jewish and Christian mysticism were composed in the darkest times of the Middle Ages. Lonely, threatened people in impersonal places may be exceptionally receptive to accepting intense parental relationships with spiritual beings. In the present day there is also increasing social dislocation, confusion, and despair. It is a fair conjecture that these conditions are major causes of the aggressive conglomerate religious identities, mystical hungering and amorphous spiritual beliefs currently distressing the world. It would be surprising if these very same conditions were not also directly affecting the healing professions that confront the distress, in much the same way as they are affecting the increasing masses of people being dispossessed of themselves.

Conclusion: religion as narcissism

At least 40,000 years ago, humans were painting the contours of spirits in cave walls and shelters and making sacrifices by inserting bone splinters into cracks in the walls, just as people still do in holy places today. They would place their palms against the walls and blow pigment on them, the imprints of which we still have. These people were seeking communion with their spirits and very probably beseeching them. About 20,000 years later, we have evidence of shamanism. The word 'shaman' means 'spirit-inspired priest or healer'.

> A shaman is a person … who has mastered spirits and who can at will introduce them into his own body. Often, in fact, he permanently incarnates these spirits and can control their manifestations, going into controlled states of trance in appropriate circumstances … It is in fact by his power over the spirits which he incarnates that the shaman is able to treat and control afflictions caused by pathogenic spirits in others.
>
> (Lewis 2003, 35)

A shaman may be fully possessed in ecstasy, or his soul may leave his body and in a nether place converse with other spirits and receive guidance. The shaman mediates between the social world and the supernatural world. Shamanistic possession, according to Lewis, is an assertion that the powers that control the cosmos and inflict calamities on humankind can be mastered; for the shaman is also powerful, god-like, living in the radiance of higher powers, conversing intimately with them, much as some televangelists, religious and spiritual people, and even psychoanalysts claim to do today.

Spirit possession is not restricted to shamans, of course. In many places where ecstatic expressions of religion are found the 'victims' of possession are often women in patriarchal societies and subordinate males with little opportunity for openly expressing their desires. The resemblances to Pentecostal phenomena of being 'slain in the spirit', speaking in tongues, and some hysterical conditions need not be pressed. Here too possession is a response to inimical circumstances which people cannot 'combat or control except through those heroic flights of ecstasy by which they seek to demonstrate that they are the equals of the gods'. 'What is proclaimed is not merely that God is with us, but that He is in us' (Lewis 2003, 30, 183). To have God or the spirits within, in the logic of the unconscious, is to have eaten them, is to be them. Identifying with powerful spirits, living in their orbits, devising mystical techniques for communing with them are defenses against helplessness and abandonment. They are methods utilizing omnipotent phantasy for regulating the narcissistic economy.[4]

It seems probable that the mystical traditions of India and the West are direct descendants of central Asian shamanism (Dodds 1951). Pythagoras, Empedocles and whoever bore the name 'Orpheus' were shamans. The various techniques of meditation, ascetic practice and mystical accession may be refined versions of shamanistic techniques for achieving ecstatic states, divesting the soul of the body and entering supernatural worlds filled with gods and spirits. In this light, most, perhaps all, mystical and spiritual experience can be understood as the initiate's short path, not only to ultimate reality, but to apotheosis. Living in communion with the gods is like being a god, near enough. The long path to reality involves the slow, difficult, piecemeal work of empirical investigation.

Notes

1 For a sober assessment of these matters, see Horton 1997.
2 The Christian background of Nazism is discussed in Pataki 2024, Chapter 8, where references are provided.
3 In 2016 and 2020 over 80% of white evangelicals voted for Trump. He is the televangelist President, a prosperity preacher whose rallies are modelled on tent revivals. An unlikely instrument of God, led to Christ by Paula White his spiritual adviser. She declared: 'I can tell you with

confidence that I have heard Mr. Trump verbally acknowledge his faith in Jesus Christ for the forgiveness of his sins through prayer'. Trump, his spiritual advisers assure us, has spoken with God and his rise was prophesied in the Bible.

4 Freud 1912–1913 and Ferenczi 1956 [1913] are the seminal discussions. Gershom Scholem's (1995 [1946]) discussion of Abraham Abulafia's mystical techniques and other elements of Kabbalistic thought are relevant in this respect.

References

References to Freud's works are to the James Strachey edition of *The Standard Edition of the Complete Psychological Works of Sigmund Freud.*

Adorno, T. W. (1950) *The Authoritarian Personality.* New York: Harper and Row.

Assmann, Jan (2010) *The Price of Monotheism.* Stanford: Stanford University Press.

Atran, S. (2002) *In Gods We Trust.* Oxford: Oxford University Press.

Bar Ness, Alice (2021) *Psychoanalysis, Mysticism and the Problem of Epistemology.* London: Routledge.

Barrett, J. L. (2007) 'Gods'. In *Religion, Anthropology and Cognitive Science,* Whitehouse, H. and Laidlaw, J. (eds). Durham, NC: Carolina Academic Press.

Bellah, Robert N. (2011) *Religion in Human Evolution.* Cambridge, MA: Harvard University Press.

Bering, J. (2011) *The God Instinct.* London: Nicholas Brearley Publishing.

Bion, W. R. (1970) *Attention and Interpretation.* London: Tavistock.

Bion, W. R. (2023 [1962]) *Learning from Experience.* London: Routledge.

Black, D. M. (ed.) (2006) *Psychoanalysis and Religion in the 21st Century.* London: Routledge.

Black, D. M. (2006b) 'Introduction'. In *Psychoanalysis and Religion in the 21st Century.* London: Routledge.

Blass, Rachel B. (2006) 'Beyond illusion: psychoanalysis and the question of religious truth'. In *Psychoanalysis and Religion in the 21st Century.* London: Routledge.

Blass, Rachel B. (2019) 'Psychoanalytic thinking on religious truth and conviction'. In *The Oxford Handbook of Philosophy and Psychoanalysis.* Gipps, R. and Lacewing, M. (eds). Oxford: Oxford University Press.

Bowlby, J. (1971 [1969]) *Attachment: Attachment and Loss* Volume 1. Harmondsworth: Penguin.

Bowra, C. M. (1973 [1957]) *The Greek Experience.* London: Sphere Books.

Broad, C. D. (2011 [1962]). *Lectures on Psychical Research.* London: Routledge & Kegan Paul.

Brown, Peter (2018 [1971]) *The World of Late Antiquity.* London: Thames and Hudson.

Capps, Donald (1995) *The Child's Song: The Religious Abuse of Children.* Louisville: John Knox Press.

Caputo, John D. (2005) *On Religion.* New York: Routledge.

Caspi, Tair (2023) 'Metaphors and the question of truth in psychoanalytic language'. In *The Routledge International Handbook of Psychoanalysis and Philosophy.* Govrin, Aner and Caspi, Tair (eds). Oxford and New York: Routledge.

Clottes, Jean (2016) *What is Paleolithic Art?*Chicago and London: University of Chicago Press.

Cockett, Richard (2024) *Vienna: How the City of Ideas Created the Modern World.* New Haven: Yale University Press.

Collins, John J. (2007) 'Israel'. In *Ancient Religions.* Johnston, Sarah Isles (ed). Cambridge MA: Harvard University Press.

Cunningham, Malcolm (2006) 'Vedanta and psychoanalysis'. In *Psychoanalysis and Religion in the 21st Century.* Black, D. M. (ed.). London: Routledge.

Damasio, A. (2010) *Self Comes to Mind.* New York: Pantheon Books.

Davidson, D. (1980) *Essays on Action and Events.* Oxford: Clarendon Press.

Dawkins, R. (2006) *The God Delusion.* London: Houghton Mifflin Company.

Dever, William G. (2006) *Who Were the Early Israelites and Where Did They Come From.* Grand Rapids: Wm. B. Eerdmans Publishing Co.

Dobbs, Trevor M. (2007) *Faith, Theology and Psychoanalysis.* Eugene, OR: Pickwick Publications.

Dodds, E. R. (1951) *The Greeks and the Irrational.* Berkeley and Los Angeles: University of California Press.

Dodds, E. R. (1965) *Pagan and Christian in an Age of Anxiety.* Cambridge: Cambridge University Press.

Dunbar, Robin (2022) *How Religion Evolved and Why it Endures.* Oxford: Oxford University Press.

Eagle, M. (2022) *Toward a Unified Psychoanalytic Theory.* London and New York: Routledge.

Eigen, M. (1998) *The Psychoanalytic Mystic.* London: Free Association Books.

Faber, M. D. (2004) *The Psychological Roots of Religious Belief.* New York: Prometheus Books.

Ferenczi, S. (1956 [1913]) 'Stages in the Development of a Sense of Reality'. In *Sex in Psychoanalysis.* New York: Dover.

Feuerbach, Ludwig (1989 [1841]) *The Essence of Christianity.* New York: Prometheus Books.

Fitzgerald, Frances (2018) *The Evangelicals: The Struggle to Shape America.* New York: Simon and Schuster.

Fotopoulou, A., Pfaff, D., and Conway, M. A. (eds) (2012) *From the Couch to the Lab: Trends in Psychodynamic Neuroscience.* Oxford: Oxford University Press.

Freud, S. (with Joseph Breuer) (1895d) *Studies in Hysteria. SE, II.* London: Hogarth Press.

Freud, S. (1900a) *The Interpretation of Dreams. SE, IV, V.* London: Hogarth Press.

Freud, S. (1901b) *The Psychopathology of Everyday Life. SE, VI.* London: Hogarth Press.

Freud, S. (1907b) 'Obsessive actions and religious practices'. *SE, IX.* London: Hogarth Press.

Freud, S. (1908d) '"Civilized" sexual morality and modern nervous illness'. *SE, IX.* London: Hogarth Press.

Freud, S. (1910c) *Leonardo DaVinci and a Memory of His Childhood. SE, XI.* London: Hogarth Press.

Freud, S, (1911c) 'Psychoanalytic notes on an autobiographical account of a case of paranoia'. *SE, XII.* London: Hogarth Press.

Freud, S. (1912–1913) *Totem and Taboo. SE, XIII.* London: Hogarth Press.

Freud, S. (1913j) 'The claims of psychoanalysis to scientific interest'. *SE, XIII.* London: Hogarth Press.

Freud, S. (1914c) 'On narcissism: an introduction'. *SE, XIV.* London: Hogarth Press.

Freud, S. (1916–1917) *Introductory Lectures on Psychoanalysis. SE, XV–XVI.* London: Hogarth Press.

Freud, S. (1918b) 'From the history of an infantile neurosis'. *SE, XII.* London: Hogarth Press.

Freud, S. (1921c) *Group psychology and the Analysis of the Ego. SE, XVIII.* London: Hogarth Press.

Freud, S. (1923d) 'A seventeenth century demonological neurosis'. *SE, XIX.* LondonHogarth Press.

Freud, S. (1927c) *The Future of an Illusion. SE, XXI.* London: Hogarth Press.

Freud, S. (1930a) *Civilization and its Discontents. SE, XXI.* London: Hogarth Press.

Freud, S. (1933a) *New Introductory Lectures on Psychoanalysis. SE, XXII.* London: Hogarth Press.

Freud, S. (1939a) *Moses and Monotheism. SE, XXIII.* London: Hogarth Press.

Freud, S. (1941d [1921]) 'Psychoanalysis and telepathy'. *SE, XVIII.* London: Hogarth Press.

Freud, S. (1954 [1887–1902]) *The Origins of Psychoanalysis.* Kris, E., Bonaparte M., and Freud, A. (eds). New York: Basic Books.

Freud, S. (1987) *A Phylogenetic Fantasy: Overview of the Transference Neuroses.* Grubrich-Simitis, Ilse (ed). Cambridge. MA: Harvard University Press.

Freud, Sigmund (2023 [1963]) *The Letters of Sigmund Freud and Oskar Pfister.* Meng, H. and Freud, Ernest (eds). Bensenville: Lushena Books.

Fromm, Erich (1973) *The Anatomy of Human Destructiveness.* New York: Henry Holt and Company.

Fromm, Erich (1978 [1950]) *Psychoanalysis and Religion.* New Haven: Yale University Press.

Fromm, Erich and Suzuki, D. T. (1993 [1960]) *Zen Buddhism.* New York: Harper and Row.

Fromm, Erich (2004 [1963]) *The Dogma of Christ.* London: Routledge.

Gale, Richard M. (1993) *On the Nature and Existence of God.* Cambridge: Cambridge University Press.

Gay, Peter (1987) *A Godless Jew.* New Haven and London: Yale University Press.

Gay, Peter (1989) *Freud: A Life for Our Time.* New York: Anchor Books.

Govrin, Aner (2016) *Conservative and Radical Perspectives on Psychoanalytic Knowledge.* London and New York: Routledge.

Granqvist, Pehr (2020) *Attachment in Religion and Spirituality.* New York: The Guildford Press.

Grotstein, J. S. (2009) *But at the Same Time and on Another Level.* London: Karnac.

Guthrie, Stewart E. (2007) 'Anthropology and anthropomorphism in religion'. In *Religion, Anthropology and Cognitive Science.* Whitehouse, H. and Laidlaw, J. (eds). Durham, NC: Carolina Academic Press.

Hanly, Charles (2023) 'Truth and psychoanalysis'. In *The Routledge International Handbook of Psychoanalysis and Philosophy.* Govrin, Aner and Caspi, Tair (eds). Oxford and New York: Routledge.

Hartmann, H. (1958 [1939]) *Ego Psychology and the Problem of Adaptation.* New York: International Universities Press.

Hartmann, H. (1964) *Essays in Ego Psychology.* New York: International Universities Press.

Harvey, Van A. (2013) Ludwig Feuerbach. In *Nineteenth-Century Philosophy of Religion.* Volume 4. Oppy, G. and Trakakis, N. (eds). Durham: Acumen.

Hopkins, J. (2012) 'Psychoanalysis, representation, and neuroscience: The Freudian unconscious and the Bayesian brain'. In *From the Couch to the Lab: Trends in Psychodynamic Neuroscience.* Fotopoulou, A., Pfaff, D., and Conway, M. A. (eds). Oxford: Oxford University Press.

Hopkins, J. (2019) 'Psychoanalysis and neuroscience' In *The Oxford Handbook of Philosophy and Psychoanalysis.* Gipps, R. and Lacewing, M. (eds). Oxford: Oxford University Press.

Horton, Robin (1997) *Patterns of Thought in Africa and the West.* Cambridge: Cambridge University Press.

Hume, David (1998 [1757]) 'The natural history of religion'. In *Writings on Religion.* Flew, Antony (ed). London: Open Court.

Jones, Ernest (1957) *Sigmund Freud: Life and Work, Volume Three.* London: The Hogarth Press.

Jones, James W. (2002) *Terror and Transformation: The Ambiguity of Religion in Psychoanalytic Perspective.* New York: Brunner-Routledge.

Kakar, Sudhir (2007) *The Analyst and the Mystic.* India: Penguin Books India.

Kakar, Sudhir (2012) *The Inner World: A Psychoanalytic Study of Childhood and Society in India.* New Delhi: Oxford University Press.

Kenny, Anthony (1992) *What is Faith?*Oxford: Oxford University Press.

Kernberg O. F. (2023) *Hatred, Emptiness and Hope.* Washington, DC: American Psychiatric Publishing.

Kirkpatrick, Lee A. (1999) 'Attachment and religious representations of behavior'. In *Handbook of Attachment.* Cassidy, J. and Shaver, P. R. (eds). New York: Guildford Press1999.

Kirkpatrick, Lee A. (2005) *Attachment, Evolution and the Psychology of Religion.* New York: Guildford Press.

Klein, M. (1975b) *Envy and Gratitude.* London: Hogarth.

Kris, E. (1952) *Psychoanalytic Explorations in Art.* New York: Schocken Books.

Lev, Gideon (2023) *Spiritually Sensitive Psychoanalysis.* London and New York: Routledge.

Lewis, I. M. (2003) *Ecstatic Religion: A Study of Shamanism and Spirit Possession.* London: Routledge.

Lewis-Williams, David (2010) *Conceiving God: The Cognitive Origin and Evolution of Religion.* London: Thames and Hudson.

McDargh, John (2017) 'The paradigm-shifting research of Ana-Maria Rizzuto: origins, strategy, reception, and horizon'. In *Ana-Maria Rizzuto and the Psychoanalysis of Religion*. Reineke, M. J. and Goodman, D. M. (eds). New York and London: Lexington Books.

McGrath, Alister (2004) *The Twilight of Atheism*. London: Rider.

Mackie, J. L. (1982) *The Miracle of Theism*. Oxford: Oxford University Press.

Martin, M. (2007a) 'Atheism and religion'. In *The Cambridge Companion to Atheism*. Martin, Michael (ed). Cambridge: Cambridge University Press.

Martin, M. (ed) (2007b) *The Cambridge Companion to Atheism*. Cambridge: Cambridge University Press.

Meissner, W. W. (1984) *Psychoanalysis and Religious Experience*. Ann Arbor: Yale University Press.

Merkur, Dan (2014) *Relating to God: Clinical Psychoanalysis, Spirituality and Theism*. New York: Jason Aronson.

Mills, Jon (2017) *Inventing God: Psychology of Belief and the Rise of Secular Spirituality*. London: Routledge.

Oppy, G. (2018) *Naturalism and Religion*. London and New York: Routledge.

Oppy, G and Pearce, Kenneth L. (2022) *Is There a God?*New York: Routledge.

Ostow, Mortimer (2007) *Spirit, Mind and Brain*. New York: Columbia University Press.

Parsons, William B. (2021) *Freud and Religion: Advancing the Dialogue*. Cambridge: Cambridge University Press.

Pataki, T. (2014) *Wish-fulfilment in Philosophy and Psychoanalysis: The Tyranny of Desire*. London: Routledge.

Pataki, T. (2019) 'Wish-fulfilment'. In *The Oxford Handbook of Philosophy and Psychoanalysis*. Gipps, R. and Lacewing, M. (eds). Oxford: Oxford University Press.

Pataki, T. (2024) *Religion, Narcissism and Fanaticism*. New York: Routledge.

Paul, Robert A. (2021) *Our Two Track Minds: Rehabilitating Freud on Culture*. New York: Bloomsbury.

Pearson, W. and Marlo, H. (eds) (2020) *The Spiritual Psyche in Psychotherapy: Mysticism, Intersubjectivity and Psychoanalysis*. London: Routledge.

Pickering, Judith (2019) *The Search for Meaning in Psychotherapy: Spiritual Practice, The Apophatic Way and Bion*. London: Routledge.

Rizzuto, Ana-Maria (1979) *The Birth of the Living God: A psychoanalytic Study*. Chicago: University of Chicago Press.

Rizzuto, Ana-Maria (1998) *Why Did Freud Reject God?*New Haven and London: Yale University Press.

Rubin, Jeffrey B. (2006) 'Psychoanalysis and spirituality'. In *Psychoanalysis and Religion in the 21st Century.* Black, D. M. (ed.). London: Routledge.

Sandler, J. (1989) 'Unconscious wishes and human relationships'. In *Dimensions of Psychoanalysis.* Sandler, J. (ed). London: Karnac.

Sandler, J. and Sandler, A. M. (1998) *Internal Objects Revisited.* London: International Universities Press.

Scholem, Gershon (1995 [1946]) *Major Trends in Jewish Mysticism.* New York: Schocken Books.

Segal, H. (1986) *Delusion and Artistic Creativity and Other Essays.* London: Free Association Books.

Solms, Mark (2015) *The Feeling Brain: Selected Papers on Neuro-psychoanalysis.* London: Karnac.

Strawson, Peter (1966) *The Bounds of Sense: An Essay on Kant's Critique of Pure Reason.* London: Methuen.

Symington, Neville (1998) *Emotion and Spirit.* London: Karnac.

Symington, N. (1993) *Narcissism: A New Theory.* London: Karnac.

Symington, N. (2004) *The Blind Man Sees.* London: Karnac.

Symington, N. (2016) *A Different Path: An Emotional Autobiography.* London: Karnac.

Tylor, Edward B. (2016 [1873]) *Primitive Culture (2 volumes).* New York: Dover Publications.

Whitehouse, Harvey (2007) 'Towards and integration of ethnography, history and the cognitive science of religion'. In *Religion, Anthropology and Cognitive Science.* Whitehouse, H. and Laidlaw, J. (eds). Durham, NC: Carolina Academic Press.

Whitmarsh, Tim (2015) *Battling the Gods: Atheism in the Ancient World.* New York: Alfred A. Knopf.

Williams, Bernard (2002) *Truth and Truthfulness.* Princeton: Princeton University Press.

Winnicott, D. W. (1965) *The Maturational Processes and the Facilitating Environment.* London: Hogarth Press.

Winnicott, D. W. (1974 [1971]) *Playing and Reality.* Harmondsworth: Pelican.

Wollheim R. (1971) *Freud.* London: Fontana.

Wollheim, R. (1993) *The Mind and its Depths.* Harvard: Harvard University Press.

Yadlin-Gadot, Shlomit (2023) 'The anxieties of truth in psychoanalytic and philosophic thought'. In *The Routledge International Handbook of Psychoanalysis and Philosophy.* Govrin, Aner and Caspi, Tair (eds). Oxford and New York: Routledge.

Suggested Reading

Dodds, E. R. (1965) *Pagan and Christian in an Age of Anxiety.* Cambridge: Cambridge University Press.

Gay, Peter (1987) *A Godless Jew.* New Haven and London: Yale University Press.

Granqvist, Pehr (2020) *Attachment in Religion and Spirituality.* New York: The Guildford Press.

Horton, Robin (1997) *Patterns of Thought in Africa and the West.* Cambridge: Cambridge University Press.

Kenny, Anthony (1992) *What is Faith?*Oxford: Oxford University Press.

Lewis, I. M. (2003) *Ecstatic Religion: A Study of Shamanism and Spirit Possession.* London: Routledge.

Meissner, W. W. (1984) *Psychoanalysis and Religious Experience.* Ann Arbor: Yale University Press.

Pataki, T. (2024) *Religion, Narcissism and Fanaticism.* New York: Routledge.

Williams, Bernard (2002) *Truth and Truthfulness.* Princeton: Princeton University Press.

Index

Note: References following "n" refer to notes.

For Product Safety Concerns and Information please contact our EU representative GPSR@taylorandfrancis.com
Taylor & Francis Verlag GmbH, Kaufingerstraße 24, 80331 München, Germany

www.ingramcontent.com/pod-product-compliance
Lightning Source LLC
LaVergne TN
LVHW021323070826
845179LV00023B/312
* 9 7 8 1 0 3 2 8 2 7 5 0 6 *